"A delightful and innovative path to the most profound truth, shared by the world's greatest healing traditions: the way through any trauma, stress, illness, or injury is to first put attention on the breath. The reader will not only understand through Dennis's inspired writing, but get to experience through numerous excellent, practical exercises how conscious and authentic breathing is the gateway to enhanced health and vitality."

—MEG JORDAN, PH.D., author of
The Fitness Instinct and founder and
editor of *American Fitness*

"It is extremely difficult to write well and truly about the healing role of breathing both in our everyday life and on the way to great self-knowledge. Dennis Lewis succeeds through a rare combination of clear-headed, practical thought and spiritual sensitivity."

—JACOB NEEDLEMAN, author of
The American Soul

"Dennis Lewis is a colleague, teacher, author, poet, and dedicated student of the breath and breathing. *Free Your Breath, Free Your Life* is not just a good book—it is a great book. It is required reading for all my students attending the Optimal Breathing School. It should be required reading for everyone."

—MICHAEL GRANT WHITE,
Executive Director, Breathing.com

"This is a truly inspiring and informative book. It is a master breathworker's book for those who wish to attain breath, and thus self-mastery."

—DR. JOY MANNE, author of *Soul
Therapy*, editor of *The Healing
Breath: A Journal of Breathwork
Practice, Psychology, and Spirituality*

Free Your BREATH, Free Your LIFE

How Conscious Breathing Can Relieve Stress, Increase Vitality, and Help You Live More Fully

DENNIS LEWIS

Shambhala
Boston and London
2004

Shambhala Publications, Inc.
Horticultural Hall
300 Massachusetts Avenue
Boston, Massachusetts 02115
www.shambhala.com

The exercises and practices in *Free Your Breath, Free Your Life* are not intended to replace the services of your physician or to provide an alternative to professional medical treatment. *Free Your Breath, Free Your Life* offers no diagnosis of or treatment for any specific medical problem that you may have. Where it suggests the possible usefulness of certain practices in relation to certain illnesses or symptoms, it does so solely for educational purposes—either to explore the possible relationship of natural breathing to health, or to expose the reader to alternative health and healing approaches. The breathing practices outlined here are extremely gentle, and should—if carried out as described—be beneficial to your overall physical and psychological health. If you have any serious medical or psychological problems, however—such as heart disease, high blood pressure, cancer, mental illness, or recent abdominal or chest surgery—you should consult your physician before undertaking these exercises.

9 8 7 6 5 4 3 2 1

First Edition
Printed in the United States of America

Illustrations by Linda Farquhar

⊗ This edition is printed on acid-free paper that meets the
American National Standards Institute z39.48 Standard.
Distributed in the United States by Random House, Inc.,
and in Canada by Random House of Canada Ltd

Library of Congress Cataloging-in-Publication Data
Lewis, Dennis 1940–
Free your breath, free your life: how conscious breathing can relieve
stress, increase vitality, and help you live more fully/Dennis Lewis.—1st ed.
p. cm.
1. Breathing exercises. 2. Respiration. 3. Health. I. Title.
RA782 .L49 2004
613'.192—DC22
2003026090

For Dasha

*And the Lord God formed man of the dust of the ground,
and breathed into his nostrils the breath of life;
and man became a living soul.*

— OLD TESTAMENT, GENESIS 2:7

Contents

THREE
The Metaphysical Breath

FOUR
Going Deeper—Practices and Meditations for Self-Exploration

APPENDIX A:
Other Core Teachings and Practices

APPENDIX B:
Helpful Breath-Related Exercises for Daily Living

APPENDIX C:
Suggested Practice Routines

Acknowledgments

Many people have been instrumental in the vision and writing of this book. I wish to express my gratitude to all of my teachers, students, and friends who have given me the opportunity to explore with them the mystery of the breath. I wish also to thank those thousands of people worldwide who have purchased my book *The Tao of Natural Breathing* and my audio program, *Breathing as a Metaphor for Living*, and have subscribed to my Internet newsletter, *Authentic Breathing News*. The feedback I have received has been both helpful and inspirational.

With great thanks to my "spiritual brother" David Hykes. The many intense exchanges and (usually) harmonic sounds that we experienced together and the Harmonic Chant and Awareness workshops and retreats that we gave together brought me a new appreciation of the relationship of sound and listening to the breath of life. As he has sung so beautifully: "time is breath just passing through."

My great appreciation to breath pioneer Ilse Middendorf, who helped me through workshops and hands-on work to understand, at least to some small degree, the importance of "the breathing spaces of the body," and whose book *The Perceptible Breath* provided some of the insights on vowel sounds that I have incorporated into my own personal work and this book.

Many thanks to my colleague Michael Grant White, "the Breathing Coach," who, through numerous enjoyable arguments and discussions, has helped me see and expand the horizons of my approach to the breath. Mike also gave me valuable suggestions during the preparation of the manuscript.

I wish to give special thanks to Carola Speads, whom I never met, but whose excellent book *Ways to Better Breathing* inspired me over time to develop Chapter One of my book on the seven self-directed ways of working with the breath. Her book contains many invaluable insights and exercises for anyone who wishes to explore breathing in a serious way.

Thanks to Dr. Joy Manne, editor of *The Healing Breath: A Journal of Breathwork Practice, Psychology, and Spirituality*, for reading an early copy of the manuscript and giving me some helpful suggestions.

Thanks also to Matt Licata at Sounds True for his invaluable help early on in the search for the right publisher, and to my literary agent Ashala Gabriel, executive director of the Marlene Gabriel Agency, for her heartfelt support for this book, and for the excellent advice she has given me.

Finally, I wish to express my gratitude to Shambhala editor Beth Frankl for responding so enthusiastically to an early version of this book and for her unflagging commitment to its publication.

Free Your BREATH, Free Your LIFE

Introduction

Few of us in today's stress-filled world breathe in a free, natural, and harmonious way. Our mostly fast, constricted breathing undermines our physical, emotional, and spiritual health and well-being, and deprives us, without our even knowing it, of one of the great joys of living on this earth: the expansive sensation of a free, easy, boundless breath that engages the whole of ourselves and connects us with all of life.

Interest in the breath has been growing rapidly over the past several years. Inspired by the influx of breath-related teachings from Buddhism, Taoism, and other traditions, and by recent research that shows the direct relationship existing between lung function and overall health and longevity,[1] a growing number of people, physicians included, have recently begun to tout the numerous health, healing, and fitness benefits of good breathing and to offer us various breathing exercises to help.

Breathing exercises, in fact, are becoming a dime a dozen these days. And so are the various breathing experts and gurus—physicians or otherwise—who would like us to believe, even though they often contradict one another, that they offer the final word on correct breathing for health, healing, or spiritual growth. Yet those of us who are students of the breath, who are actually undertaking a serious exploration of the breath of life, know in our heart of hearts that breathing, like living, is both a miracle and a mystery. As Hazrat

Inayat Khan says, "Life's mystery lies in the breath." The manifestations of this mystery are, indeed, myriad and boundless.

The question of what constitutes healthy breathing can be a confusing one, with many different theories and approaches, some of which are so simplistic as to be virtually useless. Some so-called breathing experts, for example, tell us that we should breathe only with the diaphragm and that if the chest expands during inhalation we are breathing incorrectly. In offering us a simple test to determine whether we are breathing "correctly," for instance, one well-known breathing expert, who in fact offers a great deal of valuable information about many aspects of breathing, tells us to put one hand on our belly and the other on our chest. He then says, "If the hand on your chest is virtually still, and the hand on your abdomen moves out when you inhale and moves in when you exhale, then you are breathing correctly."[2]

Though I am a great proponent of diaphragmatic breathing and have written at length in my book *The Tao of Natural Breathing* about the importance of the movement of the abdomen in the efficient functioning of the diaphragm, this so-called test for correct breathing is at best not very helpful and at worst very misleading. As you will see as you work with the practices in this book, healthy breathing involves the entire body. It is the capability of both our primary and our secondary breathing muscles to move in a full, free, and coordinated way[3] that enables us to gain the maximum benefit from each breath in accordance with the needs of the moment. It is the full, free, harmonious movements of all of our breathing muscles— as well as the many muscles that connect to or influence our breathing muscles—that, among other benefits, help ensure optimal oxygenation of our cells, pump the disease-fighting lymph through our lymphatic system and return venous blood to our lungs and heart, promote the health of our internal organs, turn on our stress-busting parasympathetic nervous system, and support the dynamic, overall sensation of ourselves living in the present moment.

The harmonious movements of our breathing muscles depend in

large part on the way we engage with our everyday lives, since, ultimately, all our muscles and bodily structures have an impact on our breathing. To sit, stand, move, sense, think, feel, perceive, act, and vocalize in ways that support healthy breathing, we need to increase our internal awareness, our ability to experience the sensations and energies of the body both at rest and in movement, and to see how abnormal and unnecessary tensions in our mind and body constrict our breath and our lives at every level. Many of us may find that taking up such disciplines as qigong (chi kung), yoga, and taiji (t'ai chi) can be a big help here. We may also find that going to massage therapists, Feldenkrais or Alexander practitioners, osteopaths, chiropractors, and other somatic workers can be beneficial, especially for those of us with major postural or other somatic problems.

There are, of course, *principles* of healthy breathing and living. But these principles will manifest in various ways depending on the specific physical and psychological needs and circumstances of each individual. When it comes to breathing, one size does not fit all. As you will see, there is no one set of breathing exercises or practices that is appropriate for everyone.

Because of all the confusion and contradictory assertions (and sometimes bad advice) about breathing and breathing exercises today, even by medical professionals, what is needed, I believe, is a clear, exploratory understanding of the various ways that one can work with one's breathing. I am not talking here about an understanding of brand-name personalities and schools, which come and go, but rather of the potential ways of engaging one's own intention, intelligence, and awareness in a serious exploration of the breath.

In *The Tao of Natural Breathing*, my first book on breathing, I explored some of the fundamental principles of full, free natural breathing. *Free Your Breath, Free Your Life*[4] continues this exploration with more recent insights and discoveries that have emerged from my on-going research, from working with others individually and in workshops, and from my own personal practice.

As usual, of course, I have discovered little that is new. What I believe I have done, with the help of experimentation, personal experience, pondering, and practice, as well as of the people and books listed in Acknowledgments and For Further Exploration, is found a way to organize some important principles of and approaches to breathing work that will enable you, the reader, to become your own student and guide in an ongoing exploration of your own breath. It is important to remember, however, that work with breath is, thankfully, a work that is never finished as long as we are still alive.

It is certainly true that we all need the help of teachers and practitioners who know and understand more than we do. With regard to breathing in a more natural and spontaneous way to promote health, healing, or spiritual growth, we may even need hands-on bodywork or breath therapy to deal with major physical obstacles or problems. We may also need help from others to work more deeply and intelligently with our emotions, which, as I discussed in *The Tao of Natural Breathing*, have a powerful influence on our breath. But it is also certainly true, I believe, that unless we can find a deep sustained interest in self-exploration, an exploration that includes the breath and its relationship to living and consciousness, we will not get very far no matter how much expert help we get.

Free Your Breath, Free Your Life is organized in several chapters. In Chapter One, Ways of Working with Your Breath, I attempt to shed light on the different ways of working with the breath by discussing what I refer to as the seven basic categories of self-directed breathing work. Not only do I discuss some of the main principles underlying each category, but I also offer some simple practices in each category to show how you can begin to work with your own breathing in a safe, creative way. These practices, however, are just the beginning. It is my hope that with the understanding you gain here and in the later sections of the book, as well as through the resources I list in For Further Exploration, you will be able to use the principles discussed in this section to discover and even create new practices for yourself that are relevant to your situation.

Chapter Two, Opening Up the Breathing Spaces of the Body, builds on the various approaches discussed in Chapter One to provide a simple, effective series of practices that you can undertake on a daily basis to help experience and open the basic breathing spaces of your body. It is through opening these breathing spaces that you can begin to regain the full expansive power of your breath. Once you have experimented with these practices you will be able to modify them or add other exercises based on your own individual needs.

Of course, it is not enough just to do breath-related practices, however helpful they may be. You also need to have a sense of the bigger picture. Chapter Three, The Metaphysical Breath, explores some of the psychological, metaphorical, and metaphysical dimensions of breathing, especially the impact of our self-image on our breathing and the relationship of exhalation to letting go. You will learn how many of the manifestations of your self-image—including the clothes you wear, the perfumes or aftershaves you use, the way you work out, and your sense of self-importance or insecurity—all influence your breathing. You will also learn some simple, powerful practices for helping you to exhale both physically and psychologically. For if there is any fundamental secret to discovering our own authentic breath, it has to do with learning how to exhale fully, to let go of what is no longer necessary.

Chapter Four, Going Deeper—Practices and Meditations for Self-Exploration, goes deeper into the breath from a meditative standpoint, exploring some integrated practices that can support your quest for healing, self-knowledge, and self-transformation. The six practices in this section are: Conscious Breathing, The Six Healing Exhalations, The Smiling Breath, The Breath of the Heart, Expanding Time, and The Boundless Breath.

Appendix A, Other Core Teachings and Practices, includes other important core teachings, as well as auxiliary practices, including the Ten Secrets of Authentic Breathing, a discussion of the importance of breathing through your nose, suggestions on how to work with your breathing using the least effort, and a Conscious Standing Practice and a Conscious Walking Practice that you can incorporate into your everyday life. These teachings and practices are referenced within the main text when appropriate.

Appendix B, Helpful Breath-Related Exercises for Daily Living, consists of a collection of easy-to-learn breath-related exercises for working with stress, tension, pain, and anger in your daily life, as well as a simple but effective practice to help you slow down your breathing.

Appendix C, Suggested Practice Routines, offers some suggested daily and weekly practice routines to get the most from the many practices and exercises in this book.

It is important to understand that although *Free Your Breath, Free Your Life* is certainly about better breathing, health, and healing, and although it does offer many insights and practices that will help you deal with the stress-related problems in your life, it does not offer or promote specific breathing techniques for overcoming specific medical problems or for weight loss, sexual performance, voice development, and so on. Free, natural, healthy breathing—which is our birthright—is not equivalent to taking a prescription pill or going on a diet. By providing a healing pathway into the deepest recesses of our ourselves, such breathing supports our overall health, as well as our performance, at every imaginable level of our lives.

At its heart, *Free Your Breath, Free Your Life* is about inner exploration, discovery, and transformation through the breath of life itself. Many of us today feel like we're suffocating, like we just don't have enough time, space, and energy to live in a way that would make us truly happy. We often feel ourselves distracted and pulled in many directions, unable to move toward or from our own center, and unable to relate fully and freely with others. We also frequently find ourselves holding our breath in the ever-increasing stressful circumstances of our lives or breathing in fast, irregular, and restricted ways. This is no small problem. Over time, such breathing reduces the amount of oxygen reaching the cells of our brain and body. A chronic reduction of oxygen is not only instrumental in many diseases, but it also reduces our capacity to sense, feel, think, and act in clear, sensitive, and effective ways.

The way we breathe, of course, is often a revealing metaphor for our willingness or ability to experience what is actually going on inside ourselves and to move freely through and within our lives and ourselves. For some of us, for example, our restricted, superficial breathing is our unconscious way of suppressing our emotions, of feeling less. Opening up the restrictions in our breathing can help us open up the experiential spaces of our own minds and bodies and learn how to live in the full expanse of the present moment. It is in the spacious reality of the present moment that real exploration, healing, and wholeness can take place.

To live from more of the whole of ourselves is only possible, I believe, when we can fully exhale, when we can let go of everything that is truly unnecessary in our lives. We're not just talking about a physical act here; we're also talking about a psychological and spiritual one as well. Can I let go, moment-by-moment, of my narrow, illusory self-image and all the unnecessary muscular tensions and contractions that arise from it? Can I let go moment-by-moment of all the unnecessary and fictitious things, both big and small, that I get attached to and identify with, so that I can receive new, more honest and complete impressions and perceptions of myself and others? Can I live and relate from my wholeness right now instead of from my assumptions, opinions, and judgments based on past experiences and future expectations?

This is what the process of health, healing, and self-transformation is really all about—the inner space and freedom to explore, to be, and to appreciate who or what I already am in my essence. The way we breathe, the way we participate day-by-day in *the breath of life*—the boundless life force that animates and connects us all—can play a vital role in this intimate exploration.

TIPS ON HOW TO USE THIS BOOK

I suggest that you read Chapter One through Chapter Three of the book sequentially and read all the material relevant to any exercise, practice, or meditation before undertaking it. Read the teachings and practices in Appendix A when it is suggested to do so. You can read Appendix B and Appendix C at any time. When doing the meditative practices in Chapter Four, I suggest that you work with Conscious Breathing daily for at least a couple of weeks before trying whichever other practices appeal to you at the time.

In general, it is best to practice in loose, comfortable clothing in a space where you won't be interrupted. When working on the floor, be sure to work on a carpet or mat, and feel free to use cushions under your head or other parts of your body in any postures that are uncomfortable for you. If possible, work in a space where there is plenty of fresh air. For most of the practices it's best to wait at least sixty minutes after eating before undertaking them. And don't forget to turn off the ringer on your phone.

Remember to work as slowly and gently as possibly, inhaling and exhaling only through your nose unless otherwise directed (please read the discussion of why nose breathing is so important in Appendix A).

The illustrations included with some of the practices are a general guide only. Use them when necessary to help you get the general idea of the postures or movements involved, but don't try to imitate them to the letter.[5]

After you have finished a practice, give yourself a few moments to take an impression—a kind of multidimensional internal snapshot—of how the practice has affected you. This is extremely important. By maintaining awareness both during and just after a practice, you will give your brain and nervous system time to integrate both the action and the results of the action into your breathing patterns and your life.

Because many of these practices—especially at the beginning—demand a great deal of attention, don't try to do them while driving, operating dangerous equipment, or undertaking dangerous activities of any kind.

Be sure to read the Ten Secrets of Authentic Breathing in Appendix A for principles that you can begin to integrate into your everyday life. I suggest that you read these principles now and refer back to them often. Once you've completed the book, take a look at Appendix C: Suggested Practice Routines for some suggestions about how to utilize the practices in this book on a regular basis.

Ways of Working with Your Breath

OVERVIEW

Work with breathing has great power to transform our health and our lives. Unfortunately, some of us undertake breathing exercises and practices that are inappropriate, even dangerous, for us. Breathing exercises come in many different varieties, all of them with different strengths and weaknesses, and some with possible "side effects."

When we start doing breathing exercises, it is extremely important to determine whether the particular exercises we are doing are appropriate for our physical, emotional, and mental situation or condition at that particular time. Since there are many ways to understand and categorize work with breathing, making this determination in advance is not always easy. In this section, I explore one of those ways, one that I have been developing for some time and that I believe will be useful in helping you understand and evaluate the wide array of breathing exercises and work being offered today.

"Who cares about categorization?" you might say. "It's not the categories that matter; it's the practices, the experiences, and the results." And you'd be right, to a point. But you would also be wrong, since what you don't know can hurt you when you start working with your breath. The "wisdom of the body" is such that a change in one part of yourself, especially a change in breathing, often brings about unexpected changes in other parts as well—all in the name of homeostasis, the tendency in living organisms to maintain a state of chemical, physiological, emotional, and mental equilibrium, even though the particular form of equilibrium that finally emerges may not be particularly appropriate or beneficial for the long term. What's more, it's not just the exercises themselves that influence us. The way we do the exercises, especially if we use too much effort or force, can create bad breathing habits and ultimately restrict our breathing even more than when we began working with our breath.

In short, the very breathing exercises that can bring immediate benefits can also, in some cases, cause long-term problems. It is therefore crucial for anyone who is considering undertaking some kind of breathing work to understand something about the different ways of working with the breath—not so much the personalities and schools, but rather the underlying principles.

In exploring this important subject, I have found it both illuminating and efficacious to approach work with breathing from the standpoint of seven basic categories: conscious breathing, controlled breathing, focused breathing, movement-supported breathing, position-supported breathing, touch-supported breathing, and sound-supported breathing. These categories, which can sometimes overlap, are not meant to be all-inclusive but rather to give you a practical framework within which to better understand how the majority of the self-directed breathing exercises and practices being offered today actually work, and to help you choose the best exercises and approaches for yourself.[1]

In reality, many of the self-directed practices that you undertake in your work with breathing will undoubtedly combine a number of the different approaches I describe here to bring about positive results in a faster, more effective, or more complete way. Nonetheless, these different categories represent different approaches to working with the breath, approaches that can bring very different results depending on your particular situation. My descriptions of these categories are not intended to be exhaustive, but only to give you a foundation for further exploration in this book, on your own, or with the help of others. Let's begin now at the beginning, with conscious breathing.

CONSCIOUS BREATHING

Conscious breathing, also known as *breath awareness*, provides an intimate pathway into ourselves. Breath awareness is practiced in the world's great spiritual traditions—including, among others, Taoism, Hinduism, Buddhism, Islam, and Christianity—as part of an overall work of spiritual development and awakening. It is also practiced in many meditative, somatic, and therapeutic disciplines for health, self-discovery, and self-transformation. The effort to experience now and here that we are breathing beings in the face of the great mystery of existence is one of the most important efforts that we can undertake on behalf of our own physical, emotional, and spiritual well-being.

Since most of us are almost totally unaware of our breathing, conscious breathing should be the first step in any self-directed program of breathing work. By learning to be aware of our breath, by learning to follow the movements of our out-breath and in-breath consciously in ourselves without any kind of interference or manipulation, we can gain many new insights into the relationship of breathing to our own inner and outer lives. As breath pioneer Ilse Middendorf writes, "The awareness of breath movement encompasses the physical experience as well as the true nature of the self as we unfold our vital force into the outer world. It is this breath that we allow to come and go on its own which sustains the basic rhythms of our life processes."[2]

Conscious breathing not only provides a solid foundation for all the other kinds of breathing work, but it is also, in itself, transformational. Conscious breathing helps us cultivate inner stillness and presence. It also helps us be present to ourselves without judgment or analysis. Through becoming aware of how we actually breathe from moment to moment, through sensing and feeling how our breath shapes and is shaped by our emotions, our attitudes, and our inner and outer tensions, we liberate the wisdom of our body and brain to bring about subtle beneficial changes without any ego manipulation on our part. Direct internal awareness of our breath can by itself, for example, help slow down our breathing if, as is common, we are breathing too fast for the circumstances at hand, or it can help alter the length of the inhalation or exhalation in an appropriate way.

Unfortunately, many people who try to become aware of their breath do so in a way that only further undermines their breathing. This happens when people equate awareness with thought or visualization and find themselves thinking about their breath or visualizing it instead of actually experiencing it through their own inner sensation. Too much thinking about or purely mental concentration on our breathing can tighten our diaphragm and other breathing muscles and produce disharmonies throughout body and mind.

Yogis, qigong practitioners, meditators, and alternative health practitioners have known for a long time that conscious breathing can help reduce stress, increase relaxation, and decrease pain. Neuroscientist Candace Pert tells us that bringing our attention to our breathing during meditation brings many such benefits. Discussing the Buddhist form of meditation called *vipassana*, for example, she points out that such mindful breathing helps us "enter the mind-body conversation without judgments or opinions, releasing peptide molecules from the hindbrain to regulate breathing while unifying all systems."[3] The key, as we have already discussed, is simply to be present to our breathing, using our inner attention to follow our inhalations and exhalations as they take place by themselves.

An Experiment in Breath Awareness

When you experiment with the following breath awareness practice, especially at the very beginning, be sure to work no more than fifteen to twenty minutes or so at a time in quiet conditions. As you gain more experience with simply following your breath for short periods of time in quiet conditions, you will find yourself becoming aware of your breath spontaneously at other moments throughout the day when it may really be important to do so—for example, in the midst of stressful circumstances. The very awareness of your breath in these circumstances, the ability to follow your breath and observe how it is related to your thoughts, emotions, movements, and postures will, by itself, gradually transform the way you face stress and other difficulties in your life.

Sit quietly now on a chair or cross-legged on a cushion, close your eyes, put your hands together on your lap or put the palms of your hands on your knees, and simply *sense* yourself sitting and breathing (fig. 1.1). Allow the actual sensation of your entire body to come to life. Using your sensory awareness, your ability to listen from the inside, take note of your weight on the cushion or chair, the tingling of your skin, the shape and configuration of your body, any muscular tensions, and so on—all at the same time.

Within this perceptual backdrop of a kind of global sensation of yourself, just note what moves in your body as you inhale and exhale. Include the sensation of the air moving into and out of your nose, or any other sensations associated with breathing. If thoughts or feelings or judgments arise about how you could be breathing better, simply include them in your awareness and let them go—instantaneously. Don't dwell on them or act on them in any way. Don't try to improve your breathing. Just follow and sense whatever you can

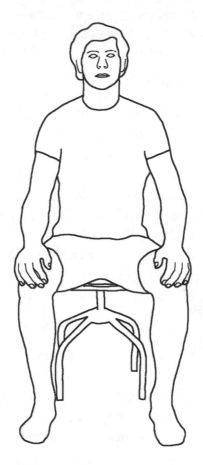

FIGURE I.I
Basic sitting posture

of your breath through all the internal sensations, movements, and pulsations of your body.

When you're ready, stop all your efforts, and simply enjoy yourself sitting there and breathing. Can you begin to sense yourself now as a breathing being?

When you're finished, just get up and do whatever needs to be done next. During the rest of the day, check in with yourself every couple of hours and note how you are breathing. Just sense and observe. Don't try to change your breathing in any way. As you become more aware of how you breathe in the various conditions of your life, of how, for instance, your breath speeds up in stressful circumstances and of how and where it tightens, or how you often unconsciously hold your breath in various emotional states, the light of awareness will by itself begin to alter your breathing in a safe, healthy, and natural way.

Later, in Chapter Four, you will have an opportunity to practice a more advanced, expanded version of this breath-awareness practice, entitled Conscious Breathing.

CONTROLLED BREATHING

When most of us think of breathing work or breathing exercises, it is generally controlled-breathing exercises that we think of. These exercises, often referred to as *breath-control exercises*, are perhaps most highly developed in the *pranayama* exercises of India and can be found in many spiritual traditions. They rely on intentionally controlling our breathing to bring about some kind of beneficial result. This result is generally brought about by altering, sometimes dramatically, the speed of our breath or the length of the inhalation, exhalation, and pauses between in order to bring about chemical, hormonal, energetic, or other changes in our body, emotions, mind, or consciousness. Controlled breathing also involves techniques such as intentional hyperventilation, fast belly breathing, alternate nostril breathing, throat locks, and reverse breathing. Many hundreds of breath-control exercises can be found in the numerous books on pranayama and yoga being offered today.

Breath-control exercises are being used increasingly by some in the medical establishment, since they can sometimes function like medications in bringing about specific chemical, hormonal, and physiological changes. Dr. Andrew Weil, for example, recounts the story of a man who used one of Weil's breath-control exercises to help reduce his blood pressure.[4] In this exercise, which Weil calls the "Relaxing Breath," one inhales for four counts, then holds one's breath for seven counts, and finally exhales for eight counts.[5] In my opinion, one of the reasons that this exercise works so well for some people is that it increases the level of carbon dioxide in the body to more normal levels (see Buteyko below), which, in this age of stress and anxiety and chronic low-grade hyperventilation, enables more oxygen to reach the cells and thus relax and slow down the nervous system.

Another doctor, Dr. Konstantin Pavlovich Buteyko, who has done a lot of research in Russia on the relationship of breathing to asthma and other medical conditions, claims that many of us have become overly sensitive to carbon dioxide in our bodies and, as a result, end up breathing "too much" in the effort to eliminate carbon dioxide and take in more oxygen.[6] As our breathing speeds up we lose too much carbon dioxide too quickly, which, among other effects, constricts our arteries and vessels and thus decreases the amount of oxygen reaching the cells of our body and brain. His solution is to breathe less; to go on what I suppose could be called a "breathing diet."[7] He prescribes specific breath-control exercises, some of which are based on breath holding at the end of the exhalation, to raise the carbon dioxide level back to normal levels.

Breath-control exercises can have many benefits if applied at the right time and in the right conditions. Leonard Laskow, M.D., for example, points out that, "Holding your breath at certain critical moments gains the immediate attention of your subconscious mind and brings your body into resonance with it through a slowing down of the heart rate."[8] He believes that by holding our breath at these critical times "we bring our body into resonance with itself, with the rhythms of the brain in its most receptive state, and with the rhythms of our planet. This synchrony greatly facilitates the reception and transfer of information and energy, both of which are critical components of healing."[9]

The Indiscriminate Use of Breath-Control Exercises

As the popularity of yoga continues to surge, breath-control exercises are becoming increasingly popular. As useful and powerful as breath-control exercises can be in well-defined situations, however, their indiscriminate use can result in harmful biochemical and hormonal imbalances, affecting not just the body but also the mind. What's more, exercises involving breath holding and muscle tensing can over time result in restrictions in our breathing muscles and tissues and undermine the harmonious coordination required for healthy breathing.[10] They can even damage the lungs through over stretching of lung tissue. As Optimal Breathing teacher and therapist Mike White points out: "Any breath-control exercise that we repeat too often will bring about restrictions in our breathing."[11] The ill effects of these restrictions may not show up for many years. It is extremely important when using breath-control exercises, therefore, to use the appropriate exercise at the appropriate time. In many cases, this will require the help of someone with more knowledge and experience who can determine the suitability of a specific exercise for the specific situation at hand.

Healthy breathing is not just a matter of the oxygen/carbon dioxide balance or other biochemical processes in the body, but is also related to the free, spontaneous rhythms and movements of breathing in our muscles, fascia, bones (including the spine), organs, fluids, and energy channels. It is the full, free, harmonious expression of these rhythms and movements of breathing that helps support our overall health and animate our being. When working with breath-control exercises that involve breath holding, throat locks, or excessive muscular tension in the breathing muscles, it is extremely important, therefore, that the practitioner already breathes (or at least is learning to breathe) in a full, natural, harmonious way.

Otherwise he or she may exacerbate any already existing problems or even create new ones.

There are, however, some breath-control exercises that are not only effective but also safe, even for beginners, and I've included a few of them in Appendix B. I suggest that you go there now to try A Safe, Simple Exercise for Stress Relief. Other helpful breath-control exercises in Appendix B that you might wish to try later include Slowing Down Your Breathing and Breathing to Transform Anger. I suggest that you don't work with these until you've reached the end of Chapter Three.

FOCUSED BREATHING

The ability to focus is one of the great powers of the human mind. Without thinking much about it, we use the power of focusing in many areas of our lives. We focus on a problem, a job, a pleasure, an aim, a person, or some other aspect of our lives. By narrowing and amplifying both our attention and our intention, focusing often enables us to perceive and accomplish much more than would otherwise be possible.

In focused breathing we use our attention, especially our sensory attention, to experience a particular area of our body, and we use our intention to direct the inner and outer movements and energies of our breath to that area. We can also use visualization to help focus on and breathe into a particular area, but it must be combined with actual sensation. When it comes to breathing, visualization without sensation can give us the illusion of understanding something that we haven't actually experienced.

Focused breathing requires no physical or emotional effort. We do not intentionally alter the rhythm or depth of our breathing. We simply *sense* (or visualize and sense) a part of our body. Then, for at least a few minutes, we allow our inhalations and exhalations to proceed *as if* we were breathing into and out of that area. Clearly, the oxygen and carbon dioxide exchange continues to take place in our lungs,[12] but we allow the physical and energetic movements of our breath to be experienced in the specific area of the body that we are working with.

Focused Breathing and Self-Healing

Focused breathing is especially useful for self-healing. The movement and energy of our breath can usually go where our attention goes, so the first step in focused breathing is to learn to be attentive to and sense specific parts of ourselves—skin, muscles, fascia, organs, bones, and so on. Because of the increased movement of tissue that it brings about in a particular area, focused breathing not only supports lymph and venous blood flow but also tissue oxygenation and much more. If we have tightness or discomfort somewhere in our body, for example, we can sometimes alleviate it (depending on its cause) by sensing the specific area and allowing our breath to engage and activate the tissues, organs, fluids, bones, and energies in the area.

Focused breathing can also help open up the various "breathing spaces" of the body, thus contributing to a fuller, more complete breath. Through breath awareness, through following our breath, we will quickly discover places in our body that are overly inflated, collapsed, or rigid, places (which could be experienced as flexible and spacious) where the alternating movements associated with inhalation and exhalation are not fully reaching. Such areas might include our belly, our lower ribs, our lower, middle, or upper back, our chest, and so on. Once we discover where we're not breathing, we can begin to focus on these areas, allowing our breath to engage them more fully.

Focused breathing can, however, cause problems. The danger inherent in focused breathing is that we may narrow our focus too much or focus too long on one part of ourselves. Such narrow concentration can further restrict the movement of our diaphragm and other breathing muscles. It can also create imbalances in our mind and body. Nonetheless, focused breathing is a powerful tool in the breathing work panoply.

Breathing into a Tight Area of Your Body

Sit quietly and scan your entire body, including your breathing. See if you can find an area in your belly, back, or chest that seems particularly tight or restricted in its movement.

Now, without using your hands or any special posture or movement, put your complete attention on that area and have the sense that each exhalation allows the area to soften and relax deeply and that each inhalation fills it with breath and energy and space. Try this for ten minutes with full awareness. Notice how you feel when you stop.

Getting to Know the Three Breathing Spaces

Sit quietly and follow all the internal and external movements of your breathing (as you did in An Experiment in Breath Awareness). Once you feel as though you are able to follow the overall movements of your breathing without any interference, pay special attention to the three basic breathing spaces of your body: the *lower space* from the navel area to the feet; the *middle space* from the navel area to the top of the diaphragm (about two inches above the very bottom of the sternum, the breastbone); and the *upper space* from the top of the diaphragm to the top of the head.

In working with these spaces, especially at the beginning, it's best if you focus primarily on the center of gravity of each space (fig. 1.2). The center of gravity of the lower breathing space is at the level of about an inch or two below the navel. This area is called the hara in Japanese and lower tan tien in Chinese. The center of gravity of the middle breathing space is at the level of the solar plexus (just beneath your breastbone). The center of gravity of the upper breathing space is at the level of the heart.

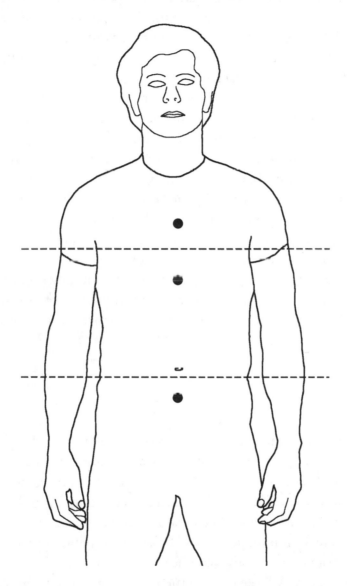

FIGURE 1.2
Centers of gravity for the three breathing spaces

Without trying to change anything, just sense the center of gravity of each space and notice how much it opens (or wants to open) with the in-breath and closes (or wants to close) with the out-breath. Work with one breathing space at a time, beginning with the lower space and moving upward after several breaths (from the hara, to the solar plexus, to the heart). Work like this for another five minutes or so. Then, taking several more breaths, see if you can sense the movements in all three breathing spaces simultaneously.

Now focus again on one breathing space at a time (starting with the lower space), but this time focus as if you are breathing only into and out of that area of your body, and have the intention that the space will expand with each in-breath and contract with each out-breath. Use only your attention and your intention. Don't use your hands or any physical or emotional force to try to open and close the space. After working a couple of minutes with each space, stop focusing and return to the pure awareness of yourself as a breathing being. Can you feel more movement in your breathing now?

MOVEMENT-SUPPORTED BREATHING

Movement is a fundamental expression of the life force. Both life and breath depend on movement. The way we breathe depends on the harmony, coordination, and fullness of the movements not only of our various breathing muscles, but also of our fascia, bones, tendons, ligaments, organs, and fluids. And these continual internal movements are in turn influenced by the outer movements that we make in the course of our daily activities.

Though we seldom think of them this way, our outer movements are for the most part automatic. Through constant repetition they have become a mostly unconscious part both of our behavior and of the way we see, feel, and sense ourselves and the world. If our movements become overly restricted in some way, as they often do because of a lack of diverse bodily challenges in our lives, our breathing will also often become restricted, with little sense of fullness, naturalness, or freedom.

For many of us, the most challenging movements we make on a day-by-day basis are getting in and out of our cars, walking to the bus stop, doing dishes, drying ourselves after a bath or shower, getting on and off our bed or sofa, having sex, changing channels on our TV remotes, and taking out the garbage. Some of us don't even get sufficient aerobic exercise to maintain a healthy heart and adequate circulation. Those of us who do have physically challenging jobs or take part in demanding physical activities of some kind often repeat the same movements over and over with little variation. Few of us are challenged to use our bodies in new, more diverse ways, so our *movement vocabulary* becomes restricted and inflexible — unable to express the fullness of the life we feel within.

Our Movements Stimulate and Shape Our Breath

In general, movement is very stimulating to breath. Each movement we make—walking, running, twisting, turning, bending, reaching, and so on—shapes our breathing in a very specific way, depending on the specific tensions and restrictions we carry in our body. Raising both arms on inhalation, for example, helps activate the breathing space in upper part of the chest and back for most people. Bending over from the waist on inhalation activates the breathing space of the lower back. Twisting in one direction or the other on inhalation helps open the breathing spaces on the opposite side of the body. Reaching straight out on inhalation activates the breathing space of the middle back. The configurations are endless.

In theory, at least, sensing the various restrictions in our chest, back, belly, and so on and intentionally undertaking a set of movements to help relax or open up these restrictions would help increase the range and power of our breath. Unfortunately, because of excessive stress, worry, fear, anger, and other negative emotions,[13] and because of excessive concentration on the "results" we hope for from our movements, many of us when we move inhibit our breathing in some way, especially at the very beginning of the movement. Holding our breath, which involves temporarily immobilizing our breathing muscles, is extremely common at the start of a movement, as is forcing our breath, narrowing it, or otherwise influencing it through mental and emotional motivations, such as anticipation, of which we are most often unaware. Thus the very movements that could help liberate our breathing often act, either directly or indirectly, only to further limit it.[14]

There are many ways of working with the power of movement to help your breathing, but they all start with breath awareness, with observing or following your breath in action throughout the day. Notice how you often interfere with your breathing when you start moving, or how your movements in various emotional states either free up or restrict your breathing. You will see, for example, that the movements you make when you are calm or happy have a very different effect on your breathing than the movements you make when you are angry or impatient—even if the movements are in your estimation more or less the same.[15]

To explore the impact of various kinds of movements on your breath, you can combine *following your breath* with specific movements designed to activate one or another part of your breathing structure. Taiji, qigong, dance, yoga, and so on can be very helpful here. You can also work with a daily program of walking (see A Conscious Walking Practice in Appendix A) and stretching. When you stretch, however, it is important that you find new, gentle, spontaneous ways to stretch. Except for certain specialized movements and exercises, it's better not to try to coordinate your breathing with your movements. Instead, just allow your breathing to adapt to the movements. This will help stimulate new, more natural and spontaneous patterns of breathing, and will give you the greatest opportunity to observe the impact of the movements on your breath.

Stretching to Open Up Your Breathing Spaces

We know instinctively how important stretching is to our sense of well-being. We feel how it can help relax our muscles, tendons, ligaments, and fascia and get our blood moving. Stretching can also help calm us down when we are anxious or fearful. As we get older, however, many of us find ourselves stretching less and less. This is unfortunate, not only for our immediate sense of well-being but also for our breathing and health.

Work with breathing is most effective when we can experience our breathing in a more intimate way. One of the simplest most practical ways to accomplish this is to observe, to sense, our breathing when we stretch. Whether we stretch automatically after sitting or standing too long or intentionally in order to explore our breath, we can begin to observe the many ways that stretching influences our breathing.

When we look closely, we will most often find ourselves inhaling as we stretch, and exhaling as we release the stretch, loosening our muscles and other tissues. This is one of the breath's natural responses to stretching. So there is no need to try to regulate the inhalation in any way when you stretch. What is needed is simply to stretch more often and more parts of yourself and to feel and sense your breathing as you stretch. It is also important in these exercises to observe your breathing for a few moments after finishing a particular stretching exercise to see how it has changed.

Stretching affects us in many ways. When I watch my Golden Retriever stretch, which she does frequently and in many ways, she seems to lengthen and expand in all directions, to stretch all her tissues, and to open up the internal spaces of her body. She especially likes to stretch while lying on her back. During the stretch she seems not only to grow longer, but also to occupy more volume. When we stretch, especially when we allow ourselves to stretch from the inside in many different ways and directions, it is possible to sense the same sorts of internal actions. As we do so, we will begin to feel the volume of our body and breath grow and expand simultaneously in several directions.

When you experiment with stretching, begin by stretching in whatever way is habitual to you. As you stretch, observe your breathing. After working in this way for a minute or two, try stretching for a couple of minutes in ways you haven't stretched before. Stretch slowly and gently with full awareness. Make sure that your stretching movements are fluid and supple. See how they affect your breath. Stretch your arms, your legs, behind your knees, your feet, your trunk, your neck, and so on. Lift your hands to the sky, push them toward the earth, twist and turn in unusual ways. Let yourself stretch from your liver, your kidneys, and other internal organs. Can you stretch from your pubic bone, your hips, your stomach, your eyeballs, your ears? Use your imagination and stretch in new ways. Just make sure that you work slowly, comfortably, and gently with full awareness.

When you are finished, take some time to sense how your emotional state and your breathing have changed. Take an overall internal snapshot of yourself. This is a very important part of the practice, since it gives your brain and nervous system time to integrate the new impressions that you've received.

The Bouncing Breath

The following practice, a version of which is said to have been practiced by Taoist sage Lao Tzu, is very useful for, among other things, reinvigorating your breath when it feels shallow and lifeless, and stimulating blood, lymph, and energy flow throughout your body.

Stand with your weight equally divided on both feet and your arms hanging at your sides. Your feet should be parallel to each other about hip-width apart (fig. 1.3a). Now take an impression of how you are breathing. Notice how much of your body is engaged in breathing. Once this is clear to you, begin bouncing up and down (letting your knees alternately bend and straighten slightly) without

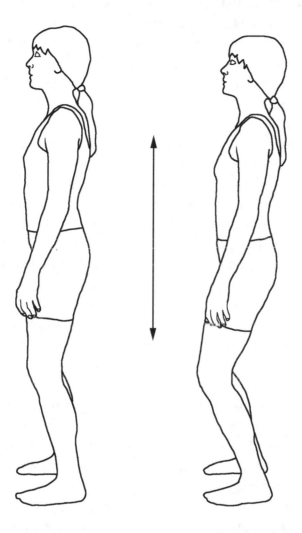

FIGURE 1.3a
Bouncing breath:
standing position

FIGURE 1.3b
Bouncing breath:
bend knees to bounce

your heels or toes leaving the floor or ground (fig. 1.3b). Make sure that your head is resting lightly on your spine and that you are looking more or less straight ahead. Start by bouncing slowly, and gradually find a comfortable rhythm that you can sustain for a few minutes. Allow the bouncing to loosen and relax your feet, calves, knees, thighs, pelvis, genitals, hips, belly, back, chest, shoulders, arms, hands, neck, face, and skull. Let it also reach and relax your internal organs.

As you continue bouncing in this rhythm, sense how your breathing begins to engage all the parts of your body. You can bounce in this way for up to five minutes at a time. When you're almost ready to stop, gradually slow the bouncing down until you feel as though you are bouncing only internally. Then just listen inwardly to your body and breath as you stand silently for another minute or so. How did the bouncing affect your breathing? What differences do you notice?

The Laughing Breath

We've known for a long time that laughter can help us heal. Recent research has shown that laughter reduces several hormones associated with stress. In fact, laughter is one of the most powerful stress-reducing tools we have at our disposal. Laughter also helps increase the level of immunoglobulin A, which helps protect us from flu and cold viruses, as well as upper respiratory problems. Laughter, especially a good belly laugh, is also a good source of cardiac exercise and promotes better breathing. Through the movements it generates throughout the body, it both relaxes and strengthens the breathing muscles in a natural way and makes them more responsive to the changing needs of our breath. It also helps clear the lungs of old air.

Try it now. To begin, take an impression of how you are breathing. Then think of something funny that has happened to you in the past that makes you laugh. Or think of a joke, a cartoon, or a fact of life that makes you laugh. If you can't come up with anything humorous enough, just start laughing at the absurdity of that rather revealing fact. Let the laugh take place deep in your belly. Laugh for at least two minutes. Then take another impression of your breathing. How has it changed?

You can also try this practice with your friends. Sit together in a room and start making funny faces at one another. Laughter is infectious, and it won't take long before you all find yourselves immersed in deep belly laughter. A few minutes of such laughter every day may well help your breathing, support your health, and lengthen your life.

POSITION-SUPPORTED BREATHING

The life force expresses itself in structural configurations of many kinds. These configurations represent each organism's way of balancing its own inherent physical form with the many inner and outer demands of living on this gravity-weighted earth. The specific positions and postures that we most often take reflect not just our needs, hopes, fears, goals, perceptions, traumas, and physical habits at any moment but also our psychophysical history and our basic stance toward living. They also reflect the degree of our openness to ourselves and others. By learning to observe our positions and postures more clearly and more often, we gain direct sensory impressions and knowledge of the forces at work in us and on us.

Every Position We Take Shapes Our Breathing

Our positions and postures, however, do more than just reflect what is happening in us. Every position and posture that we take shapes our breathing in a particular way. This fact has both negative and positive consequences. On the one hand, if we sit, stand, or lie down habitually in postures or positions that overly tighten or constrict our back, belly, diaphragm, or rib cage, these postures will over time impede the internal movements associated with healthy breathing and thus have a powerful negative influence on our breath. On the other hand, if we take a specific posture or position that helps release or open up a part of the body that is generally tight or constricted, our breathing can regain its natural coordination, elasticity, and fluidity.

Our habitual postures and positions, which represent habitual patterns of relaxation and tension throughout our bodies, obviously play a large role in the health and functioning of our muscles, fascia, tendons, ligaments, and bones, which in turn influence how we breathe. They also influence our various internal organs, as well as the way these organs are connected to one another and to the various supporting structures within the body.

In my own case, for example, my history of childhood introversion and emotional fear and insecurity, combined with many years of sitting at work slumped over at desks and computers, ultimately brought me a moderate degree of kyphosis (forward-bending of the thoracic spine) and lordosis (backward bending of the cervical spine in order to counterbalance the kyphosis), and contributed to an imbalance in the functioning of my diaphragm. This was the result not just of a somewhat collapsed chest and bent spine and unnecessary muscular tensions in my neck, ribs, and back but also of the ways in which these postures and tensions restricted the natural, spontaneous movements of my pericardium, colon, and other internal organs. As my osteopath has made clear through his hands-on work with me, the organs themselves, through their various connections with one another and the surrounding tissues, also pulled on the diaphragm and undermined its functioning. Since everything in the body is ultimately connected with everything else through influences of one sort or another, an imbalance in one place has repercussions throughout the entire organism. Osteopath Ken Lossing explains some of the complexities of these influences this way:

All the joints, organs, nerves, and tissues of the body are inter-connected by *fascia*, which is a form of connective tissue. This fascia acts like strings or cables, which can transmit mechanical tension from one part of the body to any other part. When we inhale, the lungs expand, the diaphragm drops, and all the in-ternal organs, the viscera, must move. The fascia throughout the body also moves a small amount with each breath. These movements of the organs and fascia have been shown to affect, among other things, the exchange of blood to the organs. The movements can become compromised through disease, poor posture, lack of exercise, trauma (even minor), metabolic im-balances, and emotional or physical tension. What this means from a practical standpoint is that if the attachments of the in-ternal organs to one another and to the other surrounding tis-sues are overly tight, the amount of blood and other fluids going into and out of the internal organs will be reduced. This can undermine the functioning of the organs and thus affect our health.

Recent scientific discovery has shown that the cells of the body have a substance, called *integrins*, on their walls that transmits information about mechanical tension from one cell to the rest of the cells. This information has an effect on the ex-change of fluids, gases, nutrition, and other metabolic byprod-ucts into and out of the cell. In other words, the exchanges of pressures that occur during breathing have effects all the way down to the cellular level. The better we breathe, the healthier our cells will be.[16]

Clearly, many of us have not learned to sit, stand, lie down, and move in a way that enables healthy breathing and the free movement of fascia, fluids, muscles, tissues, and so on. Many of us, for example, spend long hours bent over tensely at our desks and computers. Oth-ers of us spend long hours slumped or twisted in some way on our chairs or couches or beds watching television. Some of us do both. Such positions repeated day in and day out have a powerful negative influence on our breathing, distorting it in one way or another. Fortunately, we can, if we wish, do something about the positions and postures in which we work, play, and relax.

The Influence of Sleeping Postures on Breathing

One of the biggest influences on the way we breathe is the way we sleep. When you realize that most of us spend seven to eight hours a day sleeping, it becomes clear that the position we sleep in can have a powerful influence on how we breathe, depending on our particular body dynamics and restrictions. What's the best position to sleep in from the standpoint of our breath? There are many different viewpoints on this question, and an exploration of some of these viewpoints can be highly illustrative of some of the many complex issues involved.

Some breathing therapists and coaches, for instance, recommend sleeping on our backs. They maintain that this posture is the most efficient breathing posture since it allows the diaphragm, belly, rib cage, organs, and limbs more freedom of movement than sleeping on our belly or side. Breathing teacher and therapist Michael Grant White agrees. However, in a phone conversation with me, he pointed out that although "sleeping on one's back is the best posture for people who aspire to breathe in an optimal way or who don't have major emotional problems, it may not always be the best posture for people whose breathing is compromised in some way."

Some proponents of the Buteyko breathing approach, for example, say we should not sleep on our backs, especially if we have asthma, because this position promotes "overbreathing," which they believe dispels too much carbon dioxide too quickly, which in turn constricts our breathing airways and hinders oxygen from reaching our cells. They suggest that we should sleep on our left side. Though I do not agree that "overbreathing" is the actual problem, but only a manifestation of it,[17] it may certainly make sense for those with asthma to sleep on their left or right side until they are able to resolve the issues relating to their asthma.

There is also some recent research that points out that people who snore or have sleep apnea, especially if they are overweight, would do better to sleep on their sides than on their backs. Though many people are unaware of this, snoring and sleep apnea, which represent disruptions of our breathing, are signals of potential health problems and should not be taken lightly. People with sleep apnea, for instance, have been found to have a greater likelihood of developing high blood pressure.[18]

When we sleep on our belly, of course, we may sometimes find it easier to breathe into our back (unless it is itself very tense, which is often the case), but the twisting of the cervical vertebrae (unless our head is facing straight down as it does on a massage or chiropractor table with an apparatus for the head) can cause spinal torques that will influence not only the flow of blood, lymph, and energy but also the functioning of the diaphragm. What's more, the weight of our body will compress our belly and chest, and that in turn will reduce the movement of our breath in these areas. Sleeping on one's belly, therefore, often promotes shallow, labored breathing, which can leave us tired and out of sorts the next morning.

Some proponents of yoga recommend that we sleep on either the left or right side, in what is sometimes referred to as "the Buddha posture," with knees bent and a hand between the side of our face and the sleeping surface. One writer, for example, states that according to "yoga tradition, one should breathe through the right nostril at night, which means sleeping on your left side."[19] I have read suggestions from other proponents of yoga who state that if we are cold when we get in bed we should start sleeping on our left side, which they say activates our sympathetic nervous system and helps us get warm. Once we're warm, we're told to shift to our right side, which activates our parasympathetic nervous system, or "relaxation response," and helps us sleep more soundly.[20] Of course, sleeping on our side compresses one side of the rib cage and reduces movement on that side. If one habitually spends eight hours or so compressing one side of one's rib cage, it is easy to see how over time this reduced movement on one side of our rib cage while we sleep could manifest in our various waking postures as well.

Given all these variables, how should we sleep? Perhaps the best approach is to experiment, based on your own individual situation, to see what feels the most comfortable and helps you compensate for, or possibly even correct, any breathing problems you may have. It is important to realize, however, that the way you sleep can also be intimately related to your mental and emotional health and to any traumas you may still be carrying in your body and nervous system. If you have issues of safety or security, sleeping on your belly or side may make you feel safer and more secure, while sleeping on your back may make you feel extremely vulnerable. So there are many issues to explore. You may well find, however, that as you begin to breathe in a more complete and natural way your sleeping postures will change by themselves.

Experiment: Common, Restrictive Sitting Postures

Whatever their cause, the chronic restrictive sitting postures and positions we take in our everyday life restrict our breathing. To get a concrete sense of this now sit on a chair and let your head, shoulders, and chest collapse forward a bit, as you might when you're sitting at a desk working on your computer or writing checks. To get a real impression of the effects of this posture, feel free to overdo it a bit as shown in figure 1.4. Now, observe your breathing for several breaths. Notice how this "collapsed" posture restricts your breath. Now sit back up and thrust your chest out (but don't use too much force since you can hurt yourself) in a sort of frozen caricature of the classic military sitting posture (fig. 1.5). How does that posture influence your breath? To finish, rock on your sit bones forward and backward until you find a balanced sitting posture with your spine

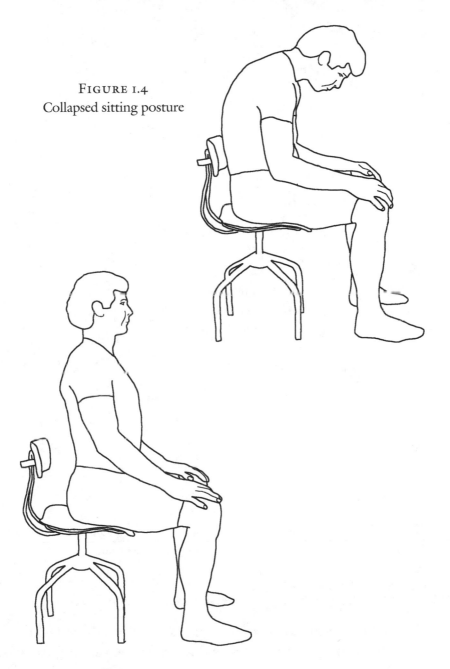

FIGURE 1.4
Collapsed sitting posture

FIGURE 1.5
Classic military sitting posture

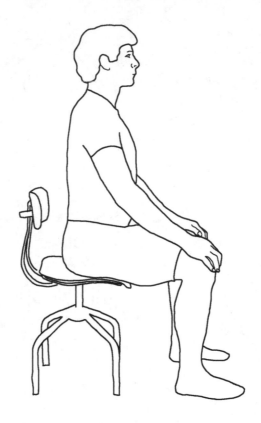

FIGURE 1.6
Balanced sitting posture

erect, neither leaning forward nor backward nor to either side (fig. 1.6). Again, observe your breath. See how it has changed.

Observe the Habitual Positions and Postures You Take

To go deeper into this important dimension of your breath you will need to begin observing how you breathe in the various positions and postures of your daily life. Notice the postures you take when you are sad, happy, bored, angry, worried, grieving, excited, and so on, and see how they influence your breath. Notice the postures you take at your desk, or watching television, talking to a friend, and other activities. See if you can observe how these postures influence your breathing.

As you work consciously in this way, you will begin to discover various, often subtle, restrictions in your breathing related to your postures. You can then experiment with new or better postures, which, by themselves, will begin to stimulate your breath to engage your body in new, fuller ways. The aim of position-oriented exercises is not, of course, only to harmonize your breathing and stimulate freer, more animated breaths (though this is, of course, often the aim), but also to give you the actual sensation of what it feels like when a particular part of your body engages in the process of breathing. Once you experience something with full awareness it is more possible to experience it again in other circumstances.

Clearly, some of the stationary postures you find in yoga can be very helpful here, as can the basic standing posture that you find in qigong (see Appendix A: A Conscious Standing Practice).

Side Bends to Open Your Rib Cage

Healthy breathing involves learning how to engage all the breathing spaces of the body: belly, ribs, chest, and back in a coordinated, harmonious way. Because of the excessive stress and tension in our lives, however, many of us have little awareness of one or another of these spaces. The first step, therefore, is to become aware of what these spaces feel like—both when they are tight and constricted and when they are more open.

For example, sit or stand now and sense both sides of your rib cage. How do they feel as you breathe? Let's assume for the moment that you find, as many people do, that your rib cage is tight on one or both sides of your trunk. Once you observe this, you can work specifically with your ribs using simple physical postures such as side bends.

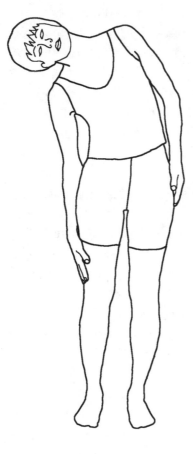

FIGURE 1.7
Bending your rib cage

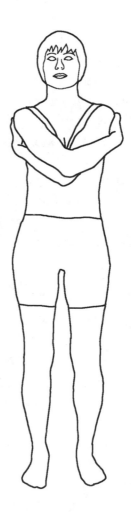

FIGURE 1.8
Hug yourself and breathe into your back

As an experiment now, either sitting or standing, gently bend from your rib cage to one side and breathe naturally in that posture for a few moments (fig. 1.7). Be sure not to thrust your hip out and don't try to breathe in any special way. Simply let the posture open up your rib cage on the side opposite to which you are bending and stimulate your breathing to expand into that area. After a few minutes, return to an upright position and sense how your breathing has been affected. Then repeat the same exercise on the other side. After a few minutes of breathing in this posture, return to an upright position again and check your breathing. Can you feel your ribs moving more effortlessly now with each breath? If not, try the exercise again. Be sure to work in a very gentle way with full sensory awareness.

Hug Yourself and Breathe into Your Back

A breathing space that many of us have a problem with is the back. Yet the back is extremely important in the process of healthy breathing, since, among other things, if it is rigid and unmoving our lungs will not be able to expand and contract in an optimal way. In a workshop that I gave with harmonic chant pioneer David Hykes, I presented a simple exercise for sensing what it's like to breathe with the back. At the completion of the exercise, one of the attendees, a singer, came up to me and said that he was amazed that he had never realized that he could breathe with his back. Here's the exercise.

Sit or stand and hug yourself by circling your chest with both arms (fig. 1.8). Grab your left shoulder blade with your right hand and your right shoulder blade with your left hand. If you cannot reach all the way to the parts of the shoulder blades closest to the spine, simply reach as far as you can. In this position inhale and exhale normally. You will notice that the pressure around your chest restricts your breathing there and automatically directs your breath into your back. Take at least nine breaths in this position, really sensing how your back begins to open and move. Then let your hands come to your sides or into your lap and notice how your back feels. Can you sense it engaging more with each breath?

TOUCH-SUPPORTED BREATHING

Most people do not realize that the skin is the largest organ system of the body, constituting about 16 to 18 percent of our total body weight and providing more than one-half million sensory fibers to the spinal cord. Many of us have a very incomplete or faulty awareness of our skin. And this faulty awareness, influenced as it is by underlying tensions in our muscles, fascia, tendons, ligaments, and so on, narrows our overall energetic sense of ourselves and impedes the overall functioning of our organism, including our breathing.

In touch-supported breathing, we use various kinds of touch to awaken and influence the sensory fibers in our skin, as well as in the areas just beneath our skin. This energetic awakening of our skin and the tissues and bones just beneath our skin can have a powerful influence on our breath, since it can help relax and release any underlying tensions. What's more, touch itself can help attract the movement of our breath. The kinds of touch we might use in our work on ourselves include gentle touch, rubbing, skin pulling, tapping, and pressure. As we shall see, each of these activities works in a slightly different way to influence our breathing.[21]

Gentle Touch

Gentle touch, especially when our hands are warm, can bring energy and sensation into an area, help sensitize and soften our tissue, and attract the movement of breath into the general area being touched. The movement of our breath likes to expand into areas where there is a sensation of comfort, relaxation, and warmth.

Rubbing and Massage

Rubbing and massage can help release tight muscles, fascia, and other tissues and thus allow the tissue to respond better to the movement of breath. By massaging our own tight belly, for instance, we help release any tension in the belly so that it can expand and contract more with each inhalation and exhalation.

Skin Pulling

Skin pulling can have an immediate and powerful impact on our breathing. In this practice, we use our thumb and fingers to grasp a fold of skin and the underlying tissue on our rib cage (especially toward the bottom or on the sides) or on our back, pull it gently away from the surface of our body, and hold it there. We can either hold the skin for several inhalations and exhalations and then slowly release it, or we can pull on the skin during each inhalation and slowly return it during each exhalation. The result of skin pulling feels rather like what happens when we take off a pair of pants that are too tight around the waist. Skin pulling gives your body more room to breathe and thus stimulates your breath to become bigger and fuller in the general area where the skin is being pulled.

Tapping

Tapping is a simple technique that can be used in a variety of circumstances. By gently tapping our skin (and the underlying tissue) with our fingertips as we sense our breathing, we stimulate the nerves in the area that we are tapping and create percussive vibrations that can travel through the muscles and help release unnecessary tensions. This can help open up any breathing restrictions we may have. The key to tapping is to tap neither too hard nor too soft on or around an area where movement is restricted. We can also systematically tap a broad area of our chest, ribs, and back. This will help release tension in these areas and help free our breath.

Pressure

Pressure is perhaps the most powerful of all touch-supported breathing techniques. It can greatly increase the elasticity of the rib cage, thus bringing about more movement in the chest and increasing the movement of the diaphragm. There are a variety of pressure techniques. In one such technique, you lightly apply fingertip pressure on a specific area of the rib cage, sternum, and back (directly on a rib, for instance, or on the intercostal muscles between the ribs). In other techniques, you can use your entire hand to apply the pressure. At the beginning, it is usually best to work on one area at a time, applying light pressure during the exhalation and gradually releasing the pressure on the inhalation. It is also important not to work too long, as this might disharmonize your breathing. There are, of course, other pressure techniques that can be used by skilled breathing therapists or teachers.[22]

The following practice, which I have taught for many years, involves a variety of the techniques just discussed. Don't underestimate the value of this simple practice. It is extremely effective.

Belly Breathing

Before we were born, our mother provided through our umbilical cord the nutrients, food, and oxygen that we needed to live. In many traditions, the area just below the navel and midway into the body is considered to be a sacred center of energy. In any event, our abdomen is one of the major areas that get tight and tense when we are under a lot of stress. And this greatly affects our internal organs, our energy, our health, and our overall sense of ourselves. It also greatly undermines our breathing.

Healthy diaphragmatic breathing is closely associated with the ability of the abdomen to expand and retract, open and close, with each breath. The extent to which the belly can move freely and easily with each breath generally mirrors the extent to which our breathing is free and natural. It also generally mirrors the extent to which we are able to be receptive and spontaneous in our lives. As breathing therapist Magda Proskauer points out, when abdominal breathing is restricted or disturbed in some way, "the inner life is disturbed; one is driven, unreceptive, and lives too intentionally."[23]

In this practice, you are going to work with belly breathing in order to open your belly and allow your diaphragm to move deeper down into your abdomen on inhalation and farther up to squeeze your lungs and support your heart on exhalation. This will have a salutary influence on the way you breathe in the many conditions of your life.

Lie down comfortably on your back on your bed or on a mat or carpeted floor. Position yourself with your feet flat on the floor and your knees bent (pointing upward). Simply follow your breathing for a minute or two with your attention. See if you can sense which parts of your body your breath touches.

Continue to follow your breathing as you rub your hands together until they are very warm. After a minute or so, put your hands (one on top of the other) on your belly, with the center of your lower hand touching your navel (see figure 1.9). Watch how your breathing responds. You may notice that your belly wants to expand as you inhale and retract as you exhale. Let this happen, but don't force it.

Above all, don't use an inanimate object such as a book on your belly, as some books on breathing suggest. Using an inanimate object on your belly will stimulate you to be more willful and aggressive in how you do this exercise, and you will lose the many benefits of using your warm, energized hands to actually attract your breath into your belly. Your breath likes to go where there is warmth and comfort, and using your hands will help create these conditions.

If your belly seems tight, rub your hands together again until they are warm and then use your fingertips to massage your belly in

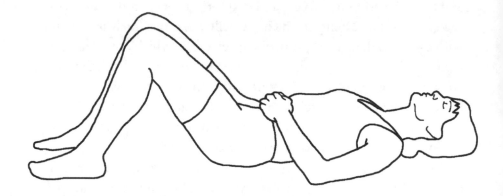

FIGURE 1.9
Belly breathing posture

small circles, especially right around the outside edge of your navel (fig. 1.10). Notice how your belly begins to soften and relax.

After rubbing your hands together again until they are warm, use your fingertips to tap your belly around (but not in) the navel. Notice how the tapping attracts your breath into your belly.

Now rub your hands together until they are warm and put them on your belly again. Watch how this influences your breath. Don't try to *do* anything. Simply feel and enjoy as your belly begins to come to life, expanding as you inhale, and retracting as you exhale.

If after several minutes, your belly still seems overly tight and does not want to move as you breathe, press down with your hands on your belly as you exhale. Then as you inhale, gradually release the pressure. Try this several times. Notice how your belly begins to open more now on inhalation and retract more on exhalation.

When you are ready to stop, be sure to sense your entire abdominal area, noting any special sensations of warmth, comfort, and energy. Spend a few minutes allowing these sensations to spread into all the cells of your belly all the way back to your spine.

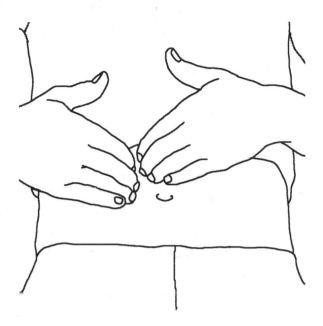

FIGURE 1.10
Massage around navel

This simple practice will have a highly beneficial effect on your breathing, especially if you do it on a regular basis. Remember that you can try this practice at any time of the day or night. Though it's easiest if you are lying down, you can also do it sitting, standing, and walking. It is an excellent practice to try before you get out of bed in the morning. It is also an excellent practice to work with whenever you are anxious or tense, since it will help relax you and center your energy. Over time, it will improve the functioning of your diaphragm and make your breathing fuller and more natural. And, perhaps just as importantly, it will give you an increasing sense of your own internal spaciousness in the midst of the many demands and pressures of your life.

SOUND-SUPPORTED BREATHING

In the beginning was the sound—the creative word of God, the colossal vibratory waves of the Big Bang, the life-giving cry of a newborn child's first breath. The sounds we produce with our vocal organs ride on the waves of our breath and contribute to the harmony or disharmony of our being, our perceptions, and our lives. They also shape the very way we breathe.

Making sustained sounds can have a powerful impact not just on our breathing, but also on our health and well-being. Most of the sounds we make involve activation of our vocal cords and take place during exhalation. Singing, humming, toning, chanting, moaning, sighing, counting,[24] and so on all influence our breath in a particular way (depending on the kind of sounds we are making and our own individual breathing habits). Over time, work with sustained or repetitive sounds can "tone" and strengthen the diaphragm and increase the height of its movement on the out-breath and the breadth and depth of its movement on the in-breath. Work with sound can also help us actually feel and give healthy expression to our often-unconscious emotions and release any negativity safely and creatively.

Each sound we make has specific energetic qualities and harmonics or overtones that touch our body, mind, and spirit in specific ways depending on our conditioning and other factors. As we sing, hum, chant, speak, and so on, the sounds and their harmonics vibrate through the surrounding tissues, bones, fluids, and energy centers and pathways, embracing and influencing everything within their range.

The sounds we make are not just the result of the activation of our vocal cords, but also of the resonance of the various breathing spaces or chambers of the body, including the belly, back, and chest. A variety of recent research shows that singing, chanting, toning, and other intentional forms of vocalization can, among other things, reduce blood pressure, heart rate, and stress hormones, and increase cell oxygenation and lymphatic circulation.[25] Some of these influences are obviously the result of a change in breathing, while others are the result of the sound's vibrations influencing the inner organs, the brain, and the nervous system. Humming, for example, apparently activates the right (more intuitive) hemisphere of the brain and helps us to relax, whereas talking seems to activate the left (more abstract) hemisphere of the brain. In fact talking often elevates our blood pressure, whereas listening generally lowers it.[26] Research also seems to show that humming can help with specific problems such as sinusitis and upper respiratory problems.[27]

The Work of Chanting, Vocalization, and Listening

In all the major spiritual traditions of the world one finds some sort of chanting—the vocalization or intonation of special sounds, words, mantras, or prayers—to uplift, to heal, and to transform. The prayers and mantras are often intoned *on a single breath*, which, among many other benefits, has the effect over time of lengthening our exhalation, increasing the strength and movement of our diaphragm, and expanding our breathing capacity.

Though it is seldom approached in this way, the Lord's Prayer is a good example of a prayer that can be chanted during a single breath. It is said to have very different physiological and spiritual effects on us when it is chanted during a single breath than when it is interrupted by the need to take another breath.[28] The sacred sound OM is a good example of a mantra that is chanted during a single breath. The ancient scriptures of both Tantric Buddhism and the Upanishads speak of the power of the chanted OM to enlighten us and free us from our karma. These traditions tell us that by chanting OM and attuning ourselves to the vibrations of pure being that it awakens, we can experience ourselves as part of the cosmic symphony.

The work with sounds, sacred or otherwise, is intimately related to meditative work, especially to the effort of listening to the vibrations and harmonics of the sounds as they resonate both inside and outside of ourselves.[29] Such work quiets and harmonizes the breath and has a calming influence on the brain and nervous system. Such work also brings us new, more global perceptions and experiences of who we are at all the various levels of ourselves. It can even bring boundless, transformative feelings of joy and happiness.

The Humming Breath

Now you're going to practice what I call "The Humming Breath."[30] Sit or stand now in an upright, relaxed posture. Let your face, tongue, and throat relax as you listen quietly to your breath for a minute or two. Then, after inhaling through your nose, exhale with the sound HUMMMM listening attentively both within your body and through your ears to the quality of the sound and the effects it is having on you. Where does the sound vibrate in you? Can you sense it in your head, face, mouth, and throat? Where else in your body can you sense it? For the purposes of experimentation, it doesn't much matter whether the pitch is high or low, only that you don't force your breath or the sound in any way. In other words, don't strain; find a pitch that is comfortable for you. When your exhalation is almost complete (when you have about 10 percent of your air left), finish exhaling without humming, and then let the inhalation arise by itself through your nose. The inhalation should be easy and effortless. Hum several times in this way.

Now, take several silent breaths sensing your belly as you inhale and exhale though your nose. Can you feel your belly expanding or wanting to expand as you inhale, and retracting or wanting to retract as you exhale? Continuing to stay in touch with your belly, begin humming again. As you hum you will sense your belly contracting inward. If your belly begins to expand outward before you have finished the sound on your out-breath, you have exhaled too long.[31] Keep sensing your belly as you take several more humming breaths, listening carefully to the quality and evenness of the sound.

Notice how the quality of the sound depends in large part on the ability of your belly during exhalation to maintain an even inward movement toward your spine. Also notice what happens with your belly as the inhalation arises by itself at the end of the sound. You will probably experience it expanding far beyond what is usual for you. Note any differences from your previous inhalations. You may be surprised at how your inhalation seems to be getting bigger— seemingly by itself.

Now take several silent breaths. Have the sense that you are breathing long, soft strands of silk in and out through your nose. When your breathing is very slow and quiet, start humming on the out-breath. This time try changing the pitch from breath to breath— but again, be sure that you do not strain in any way. After several breaths experimenting with different pitches, and once your humming has a steady, constant vibration, feel free to experiment with various vowel sounds, such as AH or OH or EH and so on. Be sure, however, to keep sensing your belly. You can work in this way for as long as you like, changing the pitch and vowels, as long as you stop making the sound before you are about to run out of breath. As you make these different sounds, notice how they influence your breath, your body, and your feelings and emotions. Whatever sounds you are making, whether humming or vowel sounds, see if you can also listen to the harmonics that are being produced, the subtler sounds above or below the main sound (the fundamental tone) that you hear.

When you are ready to stop, remain quiet for a few minutes listening to what is happening both inside and outside as you breathe only through your nose. Listen to your breath as it settles down. Notice how many more parts of your body are now engaged in the process of breathing. How do you feel? Are you more relaxed? Quieter? Just listen and take impressions of yourself as a breathing being.

In Chapter Three and Chapter Four, you will have an opportunity to experiment with other sound-oriented practices.

Two

Opening Up the Breathing Spaces of the Body

OVERVIEW

As we explore ourselves more intimately as breathing beings, we discover that the internal sensations we have of our breath and ourselves have many different densities and levels. We can discern, for example, solid, earthlike sensations; liquid, waterlike sensations; and gaseous, airlike sensations. We can experience the dense, contracted sensation of pain, the fluid sensation of ease and pleasure, and the expansive sensation of joy, love, and appreciation. We can also experience the spacious, open sensation of inner freedom—freedom from the chronic tensions and contractions of our self-image that manifest in our muscles, bones, and tissues. In this state, we begin to experience our breath and our sensation of ourselves as transparent and without boundaries.

One of the first steps in freeing our breath is learning to follow our breath through the portal of our sensation into and out of the various breathing spaces of the body. This will help us observe and release the various unnecessary tensions and constrictions in our breathing spaces. This release will enable us to breathe in a healthy and appropriate way in any situation. It will also save us an enormous amount of energy.[1]

Learning to follow our breath through our sensation is no small task. Few of us have both a global and intimate awareness of this remarkable temple of movement, sensation, feeling, and energy that we call the body. We often do not sense our internal muscular tensions and contractions—often the result of emotions such as fear, anxiety, anger, arrogance, grief, and so on—until they have already had a powerful constrictive influence on our energy and thus on our health and well-being. With each breath, however, we have a new opportunity to journey inside our bodies and, using the subtle tool of organic awareness, to forge a new, more conscious relationship with ourselves.

The following set of practices will continue to expand the work you began in Chapter One, and will help you experience and open up many of your internal breathing spaces. These practices utilize, in various combinations, all the approaches that we discussed earlier: conscious breathing, controlled breathing, focused breathing, touch-supported breathing, movement-supported breathing, position-supported breathing, and sound-supported breathing. As you work with these practices, it may be useful for you to determine which of the seven categories each exercise manifests. This will help you when it comes time to devise exercises for yourself to go further in your explorations.

Though each practice emphasizes a particular part of your body, it is important to remember that, for better or for worse, your body always functions as a whole. A practice that targets your lower back, for instance, will also affect your hips, abdomen, rib cage, chest, upper back, neck, and much more. It is important, therefore, to work with full awareness, attentive not just to the area that you are working with but also to your body as a whole. Through this subtle work of staying in touch simultaneously with the part and the whole you will gain accurate impressions of unnecessary tensions or other problem areas in your body and give your brain and nervous system the greatest opportunity to discover new, more efficient ways of functioning.

Take your time as you work through these practices. I have not designed them to be done in one session—at least not at the beginning. Work for thirty to sixty minutes at a time, being sure that you work slowly with full awareness. Once you are familiar with the practices and no longer need to look at the book in order to do them, you can undertake them all in one session. By then, you can begin to include experiments with other movements and postures and techniques as well, exploring how they affect your breathing. The key as you explore these practices is to be totally attentive to everything that is happening at the moment.

A SIMPLE EXPERIMENT WITH UNNECESSARY TENSION

We've talked about the negative influence of unnecessary tension on our breathing. Most of us, however, are unaware of our many unnecessary tensions and of the emotions that often underlie them. We've become so accustomed to them that we take them almost completely for granted, assuming that they are natural or that they are an integral aspect of who we are.

To get a firsthand idea now of how unnecessary tension influences your breathing, lie down on your back on a mat, a soft carpet, or a firm bed, with your knees bent and feet flat on the floor. If this posture creates tension in your neck, rest your head on a pillow or cushion. Be sure to breathe only through your nose. Warm your hands by rubbing them together for a few moments, then place them one over the other on your belly as shown in figure 1.9. Massage your belly gently and watch how the movements of your breath expand naturally into your belly. You may sense your belly expanding as you inhale and retracting as you exhale. Don't try to manipulate your breath in any way. Simply let yourself enjoy this sensation for several minutes. Notice how soft, smooth, and quiet your breathing becomes as it expands to include your belly.

When you are ready, get up slowly and stand in one of your ordinary postures. Watch how your breathing changes as your body begins to respond to the influence of gravity. Put your hands on your belly and just stand for several minutes. How does your breathing feel now? Experiment with different ways of standing, noticing the different configurations of tension in your body. For example, lean against a wall and observe your breathing. Can you sense how one side of your body seems to be breathing more than the other side? Experiment further. Try taking postures you associate with being anxious, angry, sad, fearful, arrogant, and so on, and see how they affect your breathing.

Now, for a minute or two each, tense and then release first your arms, then your legs, then your belly, your back, your neck, your face, and so on and notice what happens to your breathing. Take several breaths as you tense a particular part of your body. Can you notice your breath becoming smaller and tighter, with fewer parts of yourself involved? Can you notice how your breath becomes increasingly shallow, rising up higher in your chest? Then release the tension and check your breathing again.

Devise experiments of your own to see how unnecessary tension alters your breathing. If you are truly interested in learning how to breathe in a healthier way, you must take time to observe the postures and movements of your everyday life to see if they are creating unnecessary tensions that influence your breathing. We all carry unnecessary tensions in our bodies, tensions that reflect our upbringing, our stress, our frequently poor posture, our fears, our worries, our anxieties, and so on. Those of us who work at desks or with computers may begin to observe ourselves sitting with bent spines, our backs and necks filled with tension.[2] A spine that is not both erect and relaxed when we are sitting and standing greatly diminishes the free movement of our diaphragm and other breathing muscles. Once we notice these postural imbalances and tensions and see how they impact our breathing, we will understand quite clearly that healthy breathing is not just a matter of chemistry or of the right breathing techniques, but also involves sensory awareness, deep relaxation, harmonious movement, and right posture in our everyday lives.

FOLLOWING YOUR BREATH

Now that you have had a taste of how excessive tension affects your breathing, sit quietly with your eyes closed for several minutes, either cross-legged on the floor or on a chair (do not lean against the back of the chair unless you have an injury or illness that necessitates it). Be sure that your spine is erect yet supple. Your hands should be on your knees or folded gently together in your lap. As you sit, sense your weight being supported by the floor or chair, and allow the various sensations of your body to enter your awareness. See if you can find an erect sitting posture with the least amount of tension. Allow any thoughts or feelings to come and go, but do not make an "occupation" out of them.

Follow Your Breath in Stages from Your Nose into Your Lungs

Now, follow your breath as you inhale and exhale. First, sense the temperature and vibration of the air as it flows into and out of your nasal passages on inhalation and exhalation. Then continue to sense the temperature and vibration of the air as it flows into and out of your nose, throat, and trachea on inhalation and exhalation. Finally, sense the temperature and vibration of the air as it flows into your nose, through your throat and trachea, and all the way down into your lungs on inhalation, and back out on exhalation.

Take at least three or four complete and gentle breaths during each stage, and don't move on to the next stage until you can clearly sense the temperature and vibration of the air. Let the air touching these various tissues help your nose, throat, and trachea relax as much as possible. Tension in the throat, for example, which is often associated with the fear of expressing oneself, can clamp down on one's breathing as much as tension in the belly, chest, or back. Do not manipulate your breath in any way during this practice.

Sense the Expansion and Retraction of Your Belly

After at least five minutes of sensing your breath in this way, rub your hands together several times, put them one on top of the other on your navel, and sense your belly. How does your breathing respond to the warmth and energy from your hands? Can you sense your belly expanding (or wanting to expand) as you inhale and retracting (or wanting to retract) as you exhale, without losing your awareness of the entire flow of the air as it enters and leaves your lungs? Can you feel your abdomen becoming more spacious with each breath? (You may wish to try again here the Belly Breathing practice included in Chapter One, under Touch-Supported Breathing.) As your belly starts opening more with each breath, your diaphragm will move more completely through its range of motion.

Sense the Expanding and Contracting Energy in Your Belly

As you continue giving your full attention to following these movements of your breath, you may begin to have the experience of energy deep in your belly, at the level of about an inch or two below your navel. This is the area of the hara (Japanese) or lower tan tien (Chinese). During inhalation, you may feel this energy filling your expanding belly (fig. 2.1a). During exhalation, you may feel the energy becoming more compact and concentrated into this "energy center" (fig. 2.1b). Really let yourself experience and enjoy this expanding and contracting sense of energy in your belly. Continue working in this way for another five minutes or so. Then let go of the effort to follow your breathing into and out of your lungs and just come back for a couple of minutes to yourself sitting quietly.

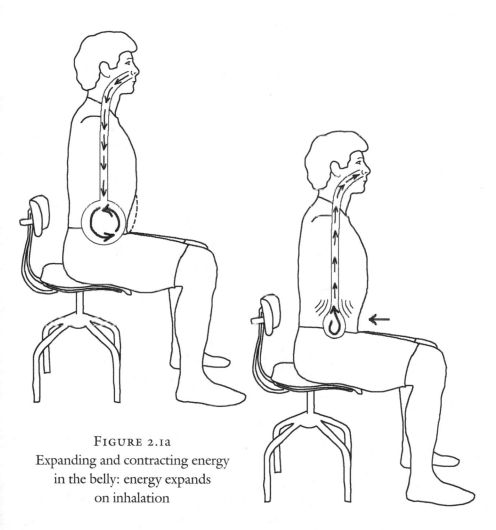

FIGURE 2.1a
Expanding and contracting energy
in the belly: energy expands
on inhalation

FIGURE 2.1b
Expanding and contracting energy
in the belly: energy contracts
on exhalation

OPENING UP THE SPACE
OF THE LOWER BACK

It is important to realize that the diaphragm is not only attached to the lower ribs, but it also has attachments to the lumbar vertebrae of your spine (fig. 2.2). This means that any tensions in your lower back will impede the smooth functioning of the diaphragm, which is your main breathing muscle. So you're going to work now to open up your lower back and spine.

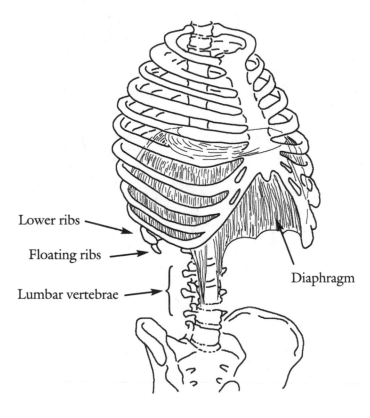

Lower ribs

Floating ribs

Lumbar vertebrae

Diaphragm

FIGURE 2.2
The diaphragm

Start with Pelvic Circles

Stand with your feet parallel about hip-width apart and your arms at your sides, palms facing back. Take a clear impression, a kind of inner snapshot, of yourself standing there, breathing. Without attempting to change anything, simply notice how you are breathing and what parts of your body your breath seems to touch or engage.

Now put your palms on the back of your pelvis, with your fingers angled downward toward your lower lumbar vertebrae, and your thumbs wrapped around toward the front of your body above your hips. When you've found a good position for your hands you should have the sense that you can use them to help control the movement of your pelvis.

Find a fixed point in the distance (looking straight ahead) and don't let your eyes stray from this point. Begin to circle your pelvis gently and slowly in the clockwise direction. Your aim is to trace a "beautiful circle" with your pelvis while keeping your head and shoulders as motionless as possible. Adjust the size of the circle until you feel quite comfortable and relaxed. If necessary, use your hands to help the movement of your pelvis (fig. 2.3).

As you continue making the circles, have the sense that you are breathing not only into your pelvis and belly, but also into your lower back. Be sure, however, not to try to coordinate your breath with the circles. Simply let your breath find its own rhythm in relation to them. After at least seven circles in the clockwise direction, begin circling in the opposite direction. Again make at least seven circles. You can then start over in the clockwise direction. Work in this way for at least five minutes. When you're finished, take further impressions of yourself standing there, breathing. See how the exercise has altered your breathing.

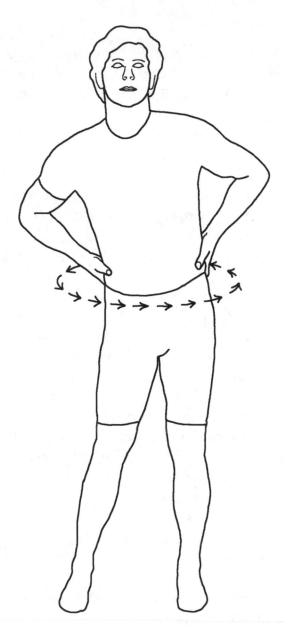

FIGURE 2.3
Pelvic circles

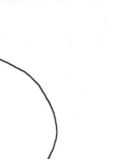

FIGURE 2.4
Relaxation pose

The Relaxation Pose

Now get down on your knees and sit back on your heels. Let your trunk bend forward until your forehead rests on the floor. Your arms should be behind, with your hands resting palms up on the floor next to your feet. In this classic yoga pose, your chest and abdomen should be pressing against your thighs, and your thighs against your calves (fig. 2.4).

Let yourself settle into this posture and check your breathing. Where do you feel your breathing taking place? As you begin to relax more completely, you will probably sense your breathing engaging more of your lower and middle back. Focus your attention on your lower back and sense how it seems to open on the in-breath and close on the out-breath. Remain in this posture for at least three minutes, enjoying this sensation of your lower back opening and closing with your breath.

Forward Bend to Open Your Lower Back

Now get up slowly and stand with your feet parallel about hip-width apart. Bend your knees slightly. Allow your head to balance lightly on your spine with your eyes looking straight ahead. Sense your weight being fully supported by the earth.

In this position, follow your breathing with your inner attention for a couple of minutes. Do not alter your breath in any way. Just sense and feel. Now, rub your hands together until they are warm and put them on your lower back. The tips of your middle fingers should be touching each other and resting on your spine just opposite your navel. Your thumbs should curl around your sides just under your lower ribs (fig. 2.5a). See how the warmth from your hands influences your breathing. Again, follow your breathing for several breaths.

Now bend forward comfortably from the point where your hands are touching your back, allowing your chest and head to hang freely, and sense how your lower back opens with the in-breath and closes with the out-breath (fig. 2.5b). After several breaths in this position, return to the upright standing position as you exhale.

Now you're going to try the bending exercise again, but this time you will coordinate the bending with your breathing. As you inhale, bend forward at the point where your hands are touching your back, focusing your in-breath in your lower back. As you exhale, return to an upright standing position. Do this several times. Bend forward as you inhale, straighten as you exhale. Sense how your lower back begins to open with each inhalation and close with each exhalation.

You can also do this entire forward-bending exercise sitting on a chair. If you do it this way, you can try it with your hands on your lower back for both the inhalation and exhalation, or you can try it with your hands sliding down your legs from your knees (fig. 2.6a) to your ankles (fig. 2.6b) as you inhale, and back to your knees as you exhale.

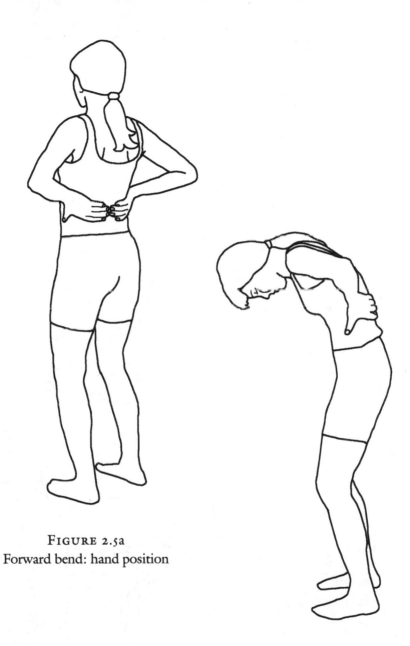

FIGURE 2.5a
Forward bend: hand position

FIGURE 2.5b
Forward bend: bend
forward at hands

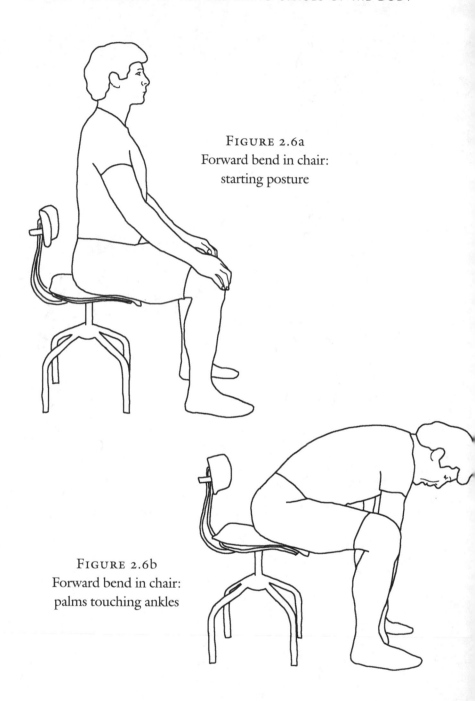

FIGURE 2.6a
Forward bend in chair:
starting posture

FIGURE 2.6b
Forward bend in chair:
palms touching ankles

Press Your Lower Back into the Floor as You Inhale

Lie on your back with your feet flat on the floor and your knees bent and pointing upward. Put your hands, one on top of the other, on your belly. Follow your breathing. See if you can sense your lower back pressing downward toward or onto the floor as you inhale (fig. 2.7a) and returning upward as you exhale (fig. 2.7b). Do not use force. Try this for several breaths.

Arch Your Lower Back as You Inhale

Now reverse the procedure. As you inhale, let your lower back arch upward away from the floor. As you exhale, sense your lower back moving toward the floor. Try several breaths in this way. (A few repetitions of this particular exercise are extremely useful for relaxation.)

Now let your lower back move toward the floor again as you inhale and away from the floor as you exhale. Take several more breaths.

Visualize a Balloon Filling and Emptying

Sense your abdomen and visualize an empty balloon inside. As you inhale, imagine the balloon filling with air, expanding your belly and pushing your lower back downward into the floor. As you exhale, the balloon empties itself, and your belly and lower back return. Try this several times for yourself.

Stop Visualizing and Simply Sense Your Breathing

Now stop visualizing and simply follow your breathing as it occurs naturally. Can you sense more movement now? If you can't, don't be concerned. Because of the sedentary conditions of modern life, most of us carry a great deal of tension in our bellies and lower backs, and it may take some time before they start to relax and open.

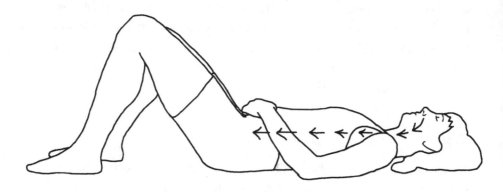

FIGURE 2.7a
Movement of lower back: in-breath

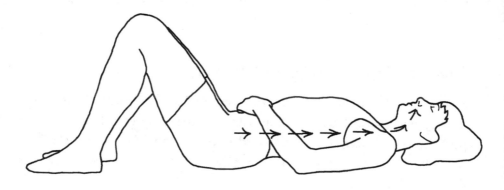

FIGURE 2.7b
Movement of lower back: out-breath

Work With the ʊ Sound to Further Open Your Lower Belly and Back

Now, as you inhale through your nose, imagine that you are making a ʊ sound (as in the word "true"). As you exhale slowly through your mouth, gently vocalize the ʊ sound. Listen to the quality of the sound internally on inhalation and externally on exhalation. Take several complete breaths in this way. Do not strain to inhale or exhale. Do not try to force air in or out. When you've reached the end of your exhalation, let the inhalation, guided by the internal ʊ sound, arise by itself. Notice how the internal ʊ sound helps to increase the sense of spaciousness in your lower belly and back and even in your pelvis. Sense how inhaling and exhaling with this sound seems to help support and ground you. Be careful, however, not to take too many breaths with this sound, as it may, if you sustain this work too long, make you feel tired or heavy. After no more than nine breaths with the sound, notice how your belly and lower back move more now with your breath.

OPENING UP THE SPACES
OF THE LOWER RIB CAGE

Earlier, we pointed out that the diaphragm is attached all around the inside of the lower ribs. When the diaphragm contracts and flattens downward on the in-breath, the ribs expand outward and swing slightly upward. These movements enable the lungs to expand and fill more completely. When the diaphragm relaxes and returns upward on the out-breath, the ribs drop slightly and return inward to their original position. These movements enable the lungs to contract and empty efficiently. It is therefore important that the lower ribs can open (and rise slightly) freely and easily during inhalation and close (and drop slightly) during exhalation. For many of us, these movements are hampered by excessive tension throughout the chest and back.

Sit on a chair now and sense your rib cage. Don't try to change your breathing in any way. When you begin to have a sensation of your rib cage as a whole, rub your hands until they are warm and then put them over your lower ribs with your fingers coming around the front of your abdomen and your thumbs reaching around the back. A good way to do this is to use your thumbs and index fingers to touch your lowest ribs, while your middle, ring, and little fingers touch your waist below your ribs. See how the warmth and slight pressure from your hands impacts your breathing. Notice how the movement of your breath begins to engage your lower ribs without any effort on your part. Can you feel them opening and closing, rising and falling?

If you find that your lower ribs are not moving at all as you breathe, press gently but steadily on your ribs as you exhale, and gradually release the pressure as you inhale. Try this several times. You can also use your fingers to massage gently between your lower ribs.

When you begin to feel your lower ribs moving, see if you can sense your belly moving at the same time—expanding as you inhale and retracting as you exhale. Work in this way for three or four minutes.

Do Side Bends to the Left and Right

Now, keeping your shoulders relaxed, let the weight of your upper body help you bend gently and easily to the left. Let your head (and left ear) also release toward your left shoulder. Try to bend as close to sideways as you comfortably can without forcing it in any way. As you do this side bend, however, be sure that you remain sitting comfortably on both sit bones (fig. 2.8). Stay in this posture for a least two minutes, sensing how the posture influences your breathing. Where do you feel that your breath is most active? Can you feel your inhalation opening more on the right side of your rib cage? Don't try

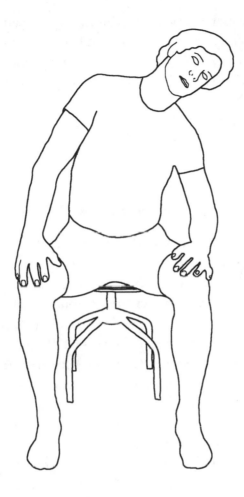

FIGURE 2.8
Side bend to left

to force this "opening" of the right side of your rib cage. Let the posture do the work.

After two or three minutes, return to the upright position and sense your breathing. Notice how the right side of your rib cage now seems to open more fully and easily with each inhalation.

Once you have this impression, bend to the right side, and put your attention on the left side of your rib cage. Again, sense how this posture influences your breathing. Where do you feel that your breath is most active? Can you feel your inhalation opening up the left side of your rib cage? Don't try to force anything. Let the posture do the work.

After two or three minutes, return to an upright position and again follow your breathing. Notice how both sides of your rib cage now expand and retract in a fuller, more effortless way.

Pull the Skin on the Lower Sides of Your Rib Cage

Now, use your right hand to grab a handful of skin (and fascia) on the lower right side of your rib cage. Pull the skin firmly away from your lower ribs and have the sense as you inhale that you are breathing into the additional space created by pulling the skin away from the ribs (fig. 2.9). Notice how the ribs on your right side expand into this space. Take several complete breaths while holding the skin away from your ribs. Then gradually release the skin back to your ribs. Take a minute or two as you breathe to notice any differences in the right and left sides of your rib cage.

Now, use your left hand to grab a handful of skin (and fascia) on the lower left side of your rib cage. Pull and hold the skin firmly away from your lower ribs and have the sense as you inhale that you are inhaling into the additional space created by holding the skin away from the ribs. Notice how the ribs on your left side expand into this space. Take several complete breaths while holding the skin away from your ribs. Then gradually release the skin back to your ribs. Take a minute or two as you breathe to notice how the lower ribs on both sides of your rib cage are now expanding and retracting more fully on inhalation and exhalation.

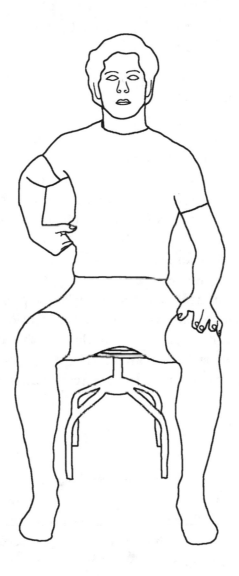

FIGURE 2.9
Skin pulling

Use the Vowel Sound A *to Help Open Up the Sides of Your Rib Cage*

Now, as you inhale through your nose, imagine that you are making an A sound (as in the word "day"). As you exhale through your mouth, quietly vocalize the A sound. Listen to the quality of the sound internally on inhalation and externally on exhalation. Take several complete breaths in this way. Don't strain to inhale or exhale. Whatever you do, don't try to "grab" your breath or to force your rib cage open. Let the internalized sound do the work. When you've reached the end of your exhalation, let the inhalation, guided by the internal A sound, arise by itself. Notice how the internal A sound helps to increase the sense of spaciousness on both sides of your rib cage. Sense how this sound on inhalation both widens and slightly lifts the sides of your rib cage. Sense how inhaling and exhaling with this sound also seems to open you to the outside world. Be careful, however, not to take more than nine breaths with this sound during any one session, as it may, if you sustain this work too long, dissipate your energy and make it difficult for you to remain calm and centered.

OPENING UP THE SPACE OF THE BACK

Now we're going to work with opening your middle and upper back. This will not only help the diaphragm move more efficiently through its range of motion, but will also allow the lungs to expand further toward the back, thus increasing their useable volume. In addition, learning to sense ourselves and our breath more from the back can serve as a powerful antidote to our growing impatience and anxiety, which directs our attention and our breath always toward the front of ourselves—into the future.

In a standing position with your arms hanging at your sides, sense your back as completely as you can. Now raise your arms above your head with your palms facing each other as you inhale (fig. 2.10), and

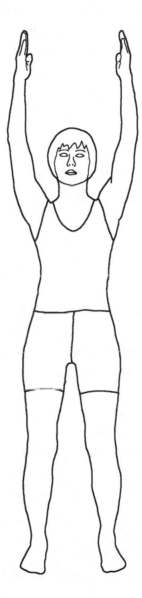

FIGURE 2.10
Raising arms above head

bring them down to your sides as you exhale. Take several breaths in this way, noticing what effect these movements have on your breathing. Now, stand on your tiptoes and try the same thing. How does standing on your tiptoes influence your breathing? How does it influence your sensation of your back?

If you would like to experiment further, you can try the exercise again, but this time exhaling as your arms go up and inhaling as they go down. Does this feel natural? How does it influence your breathing? How does it influence your sensation of your back? Finish by trying again with the arms rising on inhalation and returning on exhalation. Be sure to rest and take impressions of your breathing before continuing on.

Rocking Side to Side

Lie down on your back, with your feet flat on the floor, your knees pointing up, and your arms on the floor at your sides. Follow the movements of your breath. Notice any movements taking place in your belly, back, and chest. Are they beginning to play a larger role in the breathing process?

Now, cross your arms over the top of your chest, your hands reaching over to the opposite sides of your ribs and grabbing your shoulder blades if possible. Rock gently from side to side, using your hands to help establish the motion (fig. 2.11). Notice how this gentle, rhythmic movement relaxes your back and chest. Sense your breathing as you continue rocking for the next few moments. See if you can begin to differentiate your spine from your various back muscles. Continue working in this way until your back and chest begin to feel more open and comfortable.

Breathing Up and Down the Spine

When your back and chest feel relaxed and you can actually sense the entire length of your spine, put your arms and hands at your sides.

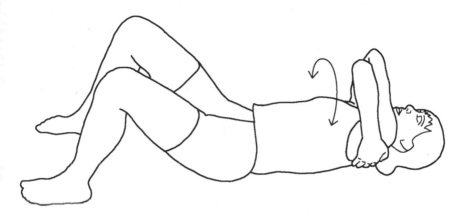

FIGURE 2.11
Rocking side to side

As you inhale, sense that the movement of your breath is beginning in your tailbone and going all the way up through your spine toward your head. As you exhale, sense the movement of your breath moving from your head downward through your spine to your tailbone. See if you can sense a subtle energetic movement along your spine as you inhale and exhale. Don't use force. Use only your intention and your attention. Work for at least five minutes sensing your breath engaging the entire length of your spine.

If you have any difficulty going up the entire length of your spine in one breath, then do it gradually, in stages, perhaps a third or fourth of the spine at a time. The important thing is to take your time and really sense the movement of your breath moving through your spine.

Hug Yourself and Breathe into Your Back

Now sit or stand and hug yourself by circling your chest with both arms, as you did in Chapter One. Grab your left shoulder blade with your right hand and your right shoulder blade with your left hand as shown in figure 1.8. If you cannot reach all the way to the parts of the shoulder blades closest to the spine, simply reach as far as you can. In this position inhale and exhale normally. You will notice that the increased pressure around your chest automatically directs your breath into your back. Take at least nine breaths in this position, really sensing how your back begins to open and move. Then let your hands come to your sides or into your lap and notice how your back feels. Can you sense it engaging more with each breath?

Try the Relaxation Pose Again

Now kneel down and sit back on your heels, as you did earlier when you did the Relaxation Pose. Let your trunk bend forward until your forehead rests on the floor. Your arms should be behind, with your hands resting palms up on the floor next to your feet as shown in figure 2.4. Once you are able to relax in this posture, focus your attention on your entire back, and sense how it seems to open on the in-breath and close on the out-breath. Remain in this posture for at least three minutes, enjoying this sensation of your back opening and closing with each breath. Then either sit or stand and sense your breathing for a couple of minutes before continuing on.

OPENING UP THE SPACE OF THE CHEST

Because so many of us already breathe mainly in our upper chests, it may be useful to point out here that no effort or force should be used to attempt to expand your chest. Though the entire chest should be able to expand and contract freely and easily with each inhalation and exhalation, the degree to which it actually expands and lifts with each inhalation should depend on the breathing demands of the moment.

Breathing therapist Magda Proskauer has this to say about chest breathing: "Normally, when at rest one breathes more with the diaphragm, like the abdominal breathing of the infant. Complete chest breathing, where the ribs expand and lift, occurs only at times of maximum effort. It usually starts the moment we pull ourselves together for action, or if we focus our attention toward outer events."[3]

Many of us today, of course, do not breathe in what Proskauer calls a normal way. Because of high levels of stress, emotional problems, tight bellies, poor breathing coordination, weak or restricted diaphragms, and many other factors, we instead try to breathe primarily using our already tense upper chests and shoulders. In fact, many people today—people who already move through life with chronically tense or raised shoulders—try to take deep breaths by raising their shoulders even more.

In a recent issue of a popular alternative health newsletter, the doctor who writes the newsletter talked about the many health benefits of good breathing. Then, in giving a detailed exercise (for filling the lungs from the bottom to the top) that he believes will help our breathing, he wrote: "Continue inhaling as the upper part of the lungs fill. As this happens, gently raise your collarbone and pull your shoulders up and back."[4]

In my opinion, though the suggestion to pull the shoulders up and back is very common, it is bad advice. Many people already carry a great deal of tension in their chronically raised shoulders and breathe mostly in the upper part of their chest and lungs, and any ongoing effort to pull the "shoulders up and back" will simply exacerbate the problem. It is not a question of manipulating the shoulders, but rather of releasing unnecessary tension and exhaling completely so that the movements associated with healthy inhalation can proceed spontaneously and unencumbered.

As you work with the following methods, therefore, don't think in terms of trying to breathe intentionally with your chest. In most cases this will be counterproductive. Let the special postures, movements, sounds, and touch-oriented techniques do the work. Your main effort should be to sense and release through awareness any unnecessary tensions so that your chest can be responsive to the needs of your breath.

Relax Your Shoulders

To prepare for working with your chest, sit now and sense your shoulders. See if you can discern any tension in them. Once you have a clear impression of what they feel like, lift them intentionally toward your ears. Hold them as high as you can while taking several natural breaths. Then let them drop and take several more breaths. Try this entire process three times. Then rotate them in circles several times forward and several times backward as you continue breathing in a natural way. Finally, just keep raising them and dropping them quickly as you take three long, natural breaths. When you're finished, sense your shoulders again and see how they feel. Notice how your breathing has changed. This is an excellent practice to undertake whenever you feel tense or anxious.

Drawing the Bow to Both Sides

There are many simple qigong postures that can help open up our breathing spaces. Drawing the Bow to Both Sides is one of my favorites.[5] As you stand, make sure that your feet are about hip-width apart. Bring your hands about twelve inches in front of your face, with your palms facing away from you and the index finger and thumb of one hand about one-to-three-inches apart from the index finger and thumb of the other hand. Your hands, which should be somewhat relaxed, will form a kind of triangle through which you look into the distance (fig. 2.12a). Keep your shoulders down and relaxed as much as possible in this position. Take several breaths, sensing what happens in your chest.

At the beginning of the next in-breath, start drawing your hands slowly to both sides, expanding your chest without effort as you make an "empty fist" (no tension) with each hand. The movement of the hands should be complete at the end of the in-breath. Have the sense that you are supporting the natural expansion of your chest on inhalation by bringing your shoulder blades together in back. Even

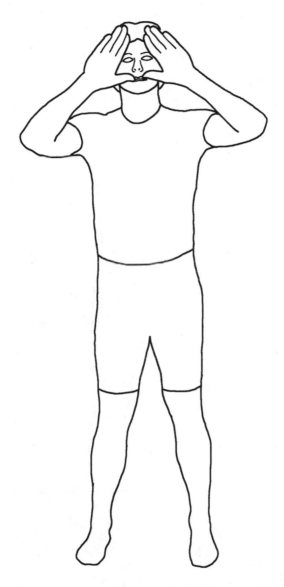

FIGURE 2.12a
Drawing the Bow to Both Sides: beginning hand position

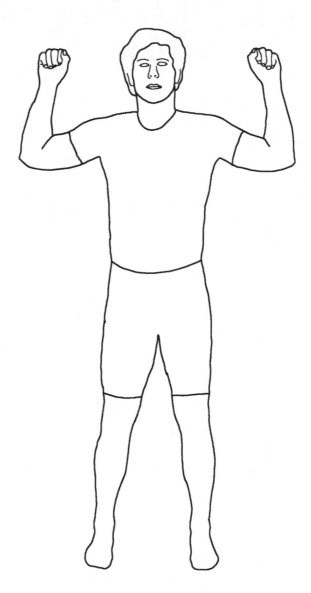

FIGURE 2.12b
Drawing the Bow to Both Sides: expand chest

though your hands are now out to the sides, be sure that they are still at the level of your eyes (fig. 2.12b). On the out-breath, the hands come back to the starting position in front of you as your chest returns to the beginning position. Have the sense that you are supporting this retractive movement of your chest by increasing the distance between your shoulder blades. Notice how these movements affect your breathing.

After at least three complete inhalations and exhalations, add the following movements. As your chest expands and your hands go out to both sides, follow the movement of your left hand with your eyes and head. As your chest retracts and the arms return in front of the face, continue following your hands back to center. On the next breath, reverse the procedure and follow the right hand as it moves. Take at least three breaths alternating in this way. Notice how the movement of the eyes and head alters your sensation of the breathing space of the chest. Before continuing, take a few moments to sense how this practice has influenced your breathing.

Using Touch and Tapping

Lie down again on your back with your knees bent and feet flat on the floor. Rub your hands together until they are warm and place them on your chest. Put your left hand on the left side of your chest, and your right hand on the right side. Your middle fingers should be about an inch apart, and the bottom edge of your hands should be touching the bottoms of your ribs (fig. 2.13). Feel the sensation of your hands on your chest and notice how this influences your breathing. You may feel your chest expanding slightly as you inhale and retracting as you exhale. Now move your hands up your chest by putting the bottom edges of your hands where the top edges of your hands were before. Your hands should be more or less in the middle of your chest now (fig. 2.14). See how your chest expands slightly as you inhale and retracts as you exhale. Now move your hands up one more time, so that the tips of your fingers are just above your clavicles

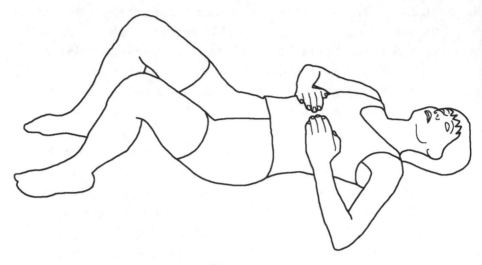

FIGURE 2.13
Hands on lower chest

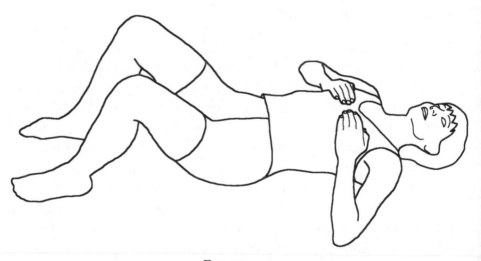

FIGURE 2.14
Hands on middle chest

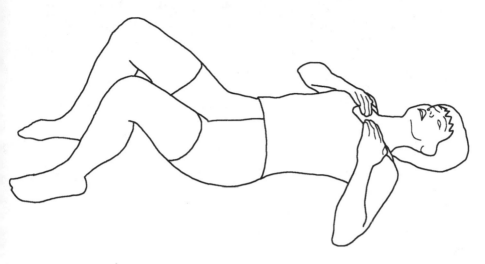

FIGURE 2.15
Hands on upper chest

at the very top of your lungs, and your palms are on your chest over your lungs (fig. 2.15). Again sense the movements of your breathing.

Now try this entire process again, this time tapping on these areas very gently with your fingertips. When you're finished tapping, put your arms at your sides and notice any differences in how your breath engages your chest.

Put Your Arms above Your Head on the Floor

Put your arms above your head on the floor, holding the fingers of your right hand gently in your left hand (fig. 2.16). Notice how this position tends to open your upper chest. Let your chest and back relax as much as possible in this open position. Take several breaths, noticing any movements in your chest and belly as you inhale and exhale. Now, reverse the position and hold the fingers of your left hand gently in your right hand. Take several more breaths and notice any subtle differences from the first position.

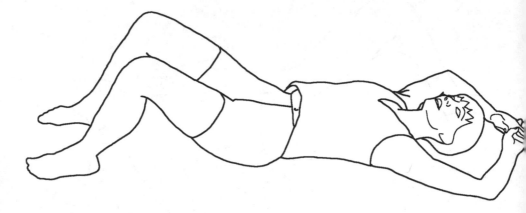

FIGURE 2.16
Arms above the head on floor

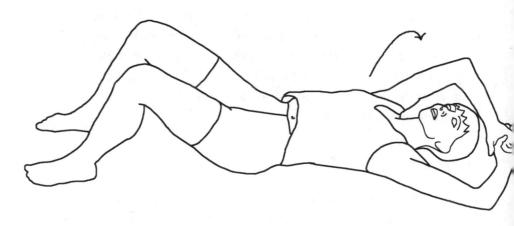

FIGURE 2.17
Raise elbow toward the sky on in-breath

Raise Your Elbow toward the Sky

Now, still holding the fingers of one hand in the other with your arms on the floor, as you inhale raise your right elbow until it is pointing toward the ceiling or sky (fig. 2.17). As you exhale, bring the elbow back down to the floor. Take several breaths in this way, sensing how these movements influence your breath. After several breaths, check to see which side of your chest seems more open with both arms above your head on the floor. Then raise your left elbow toward the ceiling as you inhale and down as you exhale. Take several breaths in this way. Again, with both arms above your head on the floor, check your breathing. Can you notice any differences?

Position with Arms in Opposition

Let your right arm remain where it is and bring your left arm down to your left side on the floor (fig. 2.18). As you continue to take several breaths in this new position, observe which side of your chest seems more open. See if you can sense the entire asymmetrical structure of your breath now. Notice which parts of your chest and belly

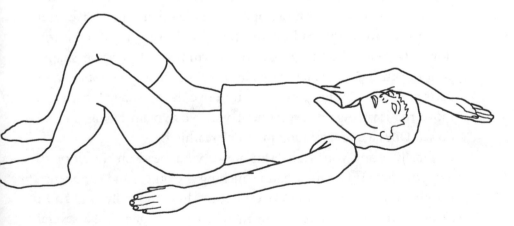

FIGURE 2.18
Arms in opposition

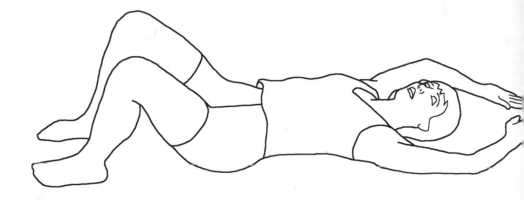

FIGURE 2.19
Arms above head

move more and which move less in this position. Experiment with the palm of your left hand facing down and facing up. Does this alter your breathing in any way?

Bring your left arm back above your head on the floor (this time neither hand holds the other). As you take several breaths in this position (with both arms above your head on the floor) notice whether one side of your chest is more open than the other. Then leave your left arm above your head on the floor, and bring your right arm down to your side. Sense how this asymmetrical position shapes your breath. Take several breaths in this position as you notice what parts of your belly and chest seem to move the most and what parts move the least. Again, experiment with your palm facing up and down. Does it alter anything in your breathing?

Finally, bring your right arm above your head on the floor to join your left arm (neither hand touching the other) and simply notice the movements taking place in your chest and belly (fig. 2.19). Does anything feel different from when you began? Take several breaths in this position, letting your chest and belly relax as much as possible.

Hug Yourself from the Back

Now sit or stand with your arms in your lap or at your side and sense any breath-related movements in your belly, back, and chest. After several breaths in this new position, hug yourself from the back. Your right hand should reach behind your back to grab your left elbow (or

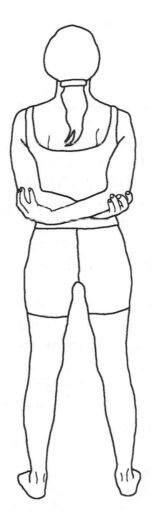

FIGURE 2.20
Hug yourself from the back

forearm if you cannot reach that far) and your left hand should reach behind your back to grab your right elbow or forearm. Keep your shoulders down as much as possible (fig. 2.20). Take several breaths in this posture, noticing whether your chest expands and retracts during inhalation and exhalation. What about your belly and back? Does this new posture help or hinder the movements of your breath in these areas? Then let your hands go to your sides or in your lap and notice how the configuration of your breath changes again.

Inhale with the o Sound

Now, as you inhale through your nose, imagine that you are making an o sound (as in the word "go"). As you exhale through your mouth, quietly vocalize the o sound. Listen to the quality of the sound internally on inhalation and externally on exhalation. Take several complete breaths in this way. Don't strain to inhale or exhale. Whatever you do, don't try to force your back and chest open. Let the internalized sound do the work. When you've reached the end of your exhalation, let the inhalation, guided by the internal o sound, arise by itself. Notice how the internal o sound helps to increase the sense of spaciousness inside your chest. Sense how this sound on inhalation both expands the chest forward and the back backward. Sense how the sound helps to bring your attention into the area of your heart. Be careful, however, not to take more than nine breaths with this sound during any one session, as it may, if you sustain this work too long, give you a feeling of disconnection or disorientation. Once you've completed this practice, take impressions of your breathing.

Raise Palm and Lift Knee

Raise Palm and Lift Knee is another of my favorite qigong exercises. It acts on one's neck, chest, back, spine, and shoulders simultaneously, and helps to release any unnecessary tensions in these areas.

Since it also includes standing on one leg at a time, it will also help you become more balanced and grounded. If you are unable for medical reasons to stand on one leg, you can eliminate the movement of the legs and keep your weight equally distributed on both feet.

Stand with your feet parallel about hip-width apart. Your right and left hands should make gentle fists, and should be placed comfortably on both sides of your waist with the palms (and fingers made into a fist) facing up (fig. 2.21a). Your weight should be equally distributed on both feet. Sense your breathing, especially in your back and chest.

Now let your weight shift to your left leg, and, gradually opening your fists, raise your left palm upward with fingers pointing backward as though you are lifting up the sky, push downward toward the earth with your right palm with fingers pointing forward, and lift your right knee until your thigh is parallel with the ground (fig. 2.21b). These movements should all begin at the very start of your inhalation and they should finish all at the same time just as your inhalation ends. As you exhale, return gradually to the starting position, arriving there just as you finish your exhalation. Then, on the in-breath, reverse the positions. In other words, shift your weight to your right leg, raise your right palm to lift the sky, raise your left knee, and push your left palm downward—all in a synchronized way.

Try this entire practice at least three times. Then, once you are comfortable with it, you can, if you wish, add the following movement of your head. As you slowly raise a palm and leg, simultaneously look slightly upward toward the sky. As your palm and leg return to the starting position, simultaneously bring your head level again. Each time you repeat the exercise, look a bit higher toward the sky, until you have reached your maximum range without creating any tension in your neck or spine. You should be able to reach your maximum comfortable range in about three more complete repetitions. If you get dizzy at any point, stop immediately, sit down, and rest. It is not necessary to add the head if it is too difficult for you to do so.

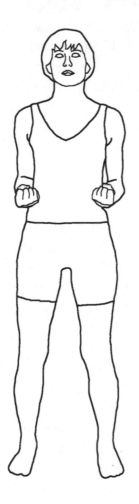

FIGURE 2.21a
Raise Palm and Lift Knee:
beginning hand position

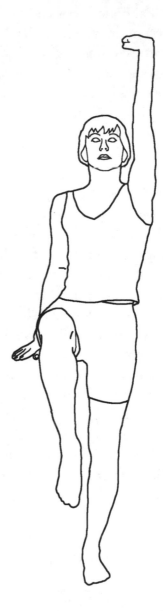

FIGURE 2.21b
Raise Palm and Lift Knee:
arm and leg positions

As you work with this practice, take your time. As soon as you feel at ease with the practice, put more of your attention on the configuration of your breathing in the various positions. Notice how one or the other side of your back, chest, and rib cage opens or closes more with each movement. Then, after you stop, check your breathing again. How has it changed?

BREATHE EVERYWHERE AT ONCE

Now you're going to return to breathing in your belly, lower back, rib cage, and back—but all at the same time. You can do this sitting or standing. As you breathe, sense any movements in these areas. Visualize a balloon or a ball of energy in your belly that expands as you inhale and contracts as you exhale. See and sense how the balloon or energy ball expands your belly, lower rib cage, back, and chest. After several breaths, stop visualizing the balloon or energy ball and simply sense the movement of opening and closing taking place in your body as you inhale and exhale. Really let yourself enjoy this increased sense of spacious movement in your breathing.

Work Alternately with the U, A, and O Sounds

To get an even deeper sense of this spaciousness, inhale and exhale for several breaths with the U sound, focusing on your belly and lower back. Then inhale and exhale with the A sound, focusing on both sides of your rib cage simultaneously. Then inhale and exhale with the O sound, focusing on your chest and back. Go through this cycle nine times, shifting your attention each time from belly/lower back, to ribs, to chest/back, and so on. Then stop making the sounds and, for several breaths, see if you can sense your belly, the sides of your rib cage, and your chest and back effortlessly expanding as you inhale and retracting as you exhale.

GETTING READY TO STOP

When you're almost ready to stop, bring your attention again to the air traveling from the tip of your nose all the way into your lungs on inhalation, and from your lungs all the way back through the tip of your nose on exhalation. Sense the warmth or coolness of the air as it touches your internal tissues. Take several complete breaths in this way.

Now, stop sensing the flow of air and give yourself a couple of minutes to sense the energy, or at least some of the energy, in your belly and rib cage being absorbed into all the surrounding tissues and cells but especially into the energy center (hara or lower tan tien) below your navel. Then bring your attention back to the whole sensation of yourself just sitting. Watch, sense, and feel everything that is taking place inside you until you are ready to stop. After you open your eyes, stretch gently for a few seconds before getting up.

SET A DAILY SCHEDULE TO GET IN TOUCH WITH YOUR BREATHING SPACES

To gain the most benefit from this set of practices, it would be helpful during the rest of the day to take a minute or so every hour or two to get in touch with your belly, ribs, back, and chest. When you try this, notice how they feel. Notice whether they are tight or relaxed. Notice whether they expand as you inhale and retract as you exhale. It doesn't matter how much they expand or contract—only that they are somehow involved spontaneously in your breath. Using your "organic memory," your body's sensory memory, compare the sensation at that moment with the sensation of your belly, rib cage, back, and chest that you had while doing this comprehensive practice. Don't analyze what you experience; simply be aware of any differences. Then continue on with whatever you need to do next.

WORKING WITH YOUR
BREATHING RESTRICTIONS

After working with these practices for several weeks, you will begin to know experientially those parts of yourself that don't participate fully in the breathing process. With this knowledge, you can spend more time opening and releasing these areas using some of the techniques in this book. If you haven't already done so, you might also wish to initiate a program of qigong or yoga that helps address restrictions in these areas. If the restrictions are particularly troublesome, it may be wise to enlist the help of a body worker, breath therapist, osteopath, Feldenkrais practitioner, or other somatic specialist. Sometimes hands-on work by an experienced practitioner is needed to support your efforts and bring about real change.

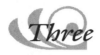

Three

The Metaphysical Breath

OVERVIEW

Now that we've explored some of the basic ways of working with the breath and have had an opportunity to try a variety of practices that illustrate them, it's important to also explore the larger metaphorical and metaphysical dimensions of the breath. It is through a journey into these dimensions of the breath that we can discover some of the conditions necessary for real transformation not just of our breathing but also of our being, our consciousness, and our life.

The great spiritual traditions of the world all have a science of breath. In most traditions, the word *breath* is related to the unknown, to the spirit, to the infinite, to the higher, subtle energy that brings us to life and enlivens us. Our breath originates from the very source of all life, whatever we may wish to call this source. In Genesis, for example, it is God who breathes "the breath of life" into man. Our in-breath represents inspiration, or creation. Our out-breath represents expiration, or death. Each breath we take can be a joyous reminder of the great mystery of birth and death and of the unfathomable energy that sustains us and enables us to unfold as individuals in space and time.

Almost every tradition equates breath with some kind of fundamental vibration or energy—an energy that can be used for healing and spiritual evolution. The *energy of breath* is related to concepts such as chi (China), prana (India), baraka (Islam), pneuma (Greece), and ruach (Hebrew) and this energy is viewed not only as the foundation of our existence on this earth but also as the vital unifying link between body, mind, and spirit. Some traditions, such as Taoism and Gurdjieff, even speak of learning how to consciously extract higher energies from the air we breathe and use these energies not just for health and healing but also for inner alchemy and even immortality. This extraction of higher energies from the air has to do mainly with the power of our inner intention and the ability to follow our breath consciously without any interference or manipulation.

In recent years, the metaphysical dimensions of the breath have not gone unnoticed by some in the medical community. In his book *Boosting Immunity*, for example, Len Saputo, M.D., is right on target when he writes:

> Breathing is much more than a simple mechanical act. Today there is a growing interest in the relationship of breathing to both health and spiritual development. All ancient indigenous healing systems consider the breath a source of life-force energy that brings healing into the body. The use of the breath is very integral to the practice of many disciplines, including yoga and Ayurveda, Taoism, Zen, and Tibetan Buddhism. Contemporary health-care practitioners are making an effort to revive these methods of breathing. These practices promote deeper relaxation and self-awareness, improved management of stress, and enhanced health and wholeness. When we are in this state of deep relaxation and the mind slows down, it is much easier to connect with spirit.[1]

As we ponder some of the vast metaphysical dimensions of the breath, we are faced with the inescapable fact that many of us in today's world breathe in a way that is narrow and constricting, a way that is unworthy of our birthright, of our inborn potential. The way that many of us breathe is detrimental not only to our physical health but also to our emotional, mental, and spiritual well-being. The traditions tell us, however—and many of us know from personal experience—that there is another way of breathing, a breath of spaciousness and freedom, what I call *boundless breathing*, that can revitalize us and support us on the path of self-knowledge and self-transformation.

Through a sustained work of self-sensing and inner awareness, we will discover that our breath does in fact go beyond what we normally think of as the purely physical, our anatomy and physiology, and reflects and embraces to varying degrees all the sides and dimensions of ourselves: physical, emotional, mental, and spiritual. We will also see that the way we live and the way we breathe go hand-in-hand. A breath that is distorted, constricted, or disharmonious in some fundamental way, a breath that is not as authentic as it can be in relation to our inborn potential, both reflects and contributes to a life that is also distorted, constricted, or disharmonious. A common example of such a distortion is the fast, primarily upper-chest breathing that is so prevalent in today's stress-filled world. According to spiritual explorer Karlfried Graf von Durckheim, such breathing reflects our "clinging, self-protecting ego," and represents "an inhibition of essential being."[2] The tight-fitting armor of our ego, our rigid and distorted self-image, constricts our body, suffocates our feelings and intuition, and hinders essential contact with ourselves and others. It blocks us from fully receiving the energies of heaven and earth—the very energies that enable us to grow and evolve.

HOW OUR SELF-IMAGE INFLUENCES OUR BREATHING

Everyone has a self-image. Everyone has a subjective identity fashioned over the years out of the material of thought, feeling, sensation, posture, and movement. For many of us, however, our self-image — which includes the conscious and unconscious sensory, emotional, and mental attitudes through which we view ourselves and others — is extremely narrow and bears little resemblance either to how others see us or to our own inborn potential. As a result, most of us live stunted or illusory lives expressing only a small part of who we really are and can be.

Our self-image — which includes our vanity, self-love, low self-esteem, insecurity, and so on — has a powerful influence on the way we live and breathe. The breathing that "nature intended for us," as Durckheim puts it, is not meant to be fixed in one place in ourselves. It is meant to embrace us in varying waves and pulsations of energy and movement. When we live in true harmony with ourselves, these waves and pulsations arise from our true center deep in our abdomen and radiate throughout our entire body. The expansion, however subtle, of the breathing spaces of our belly, back, and chest on inhalation and their retraction on exhalation help enable the diaphragm to move freely through its entire range of movement downward on inhalation and upward on exhalation. Unfortunately, the distorted, illusory way that we perceive ourselves and live often restricts this alternating movement of expansion and contraction. Though we may not notice the adverse effects of these restrictions when we're in our twenties and thirties and still bubbling over with energy, we may start noticing them as we move into our forties and fifties and beyond as our armor tightens, our breath diminishes, and our life force and recuperative powers begin to wane.

Overly Tight Clothing

Our self-image influences our breathing in a variety of ways, many of which we give little attention to. Much of the clothing that we wear, for instance, especially the overly tight clothing that some of us wear to show off our physical assets or demonstrate our Fashion IQ can greatly hamper our breathing. Tight, armorlike clothing stimulates the sensory nerves and stretch receptors in our muscles, organs, joints, and skin to send messages to our brain and nervous system to reduce movement.

Overly tight jeans, for example, as sexy as they often are, can in some cases undermine the natural movements of the pelvis and lower abdomen, and not only restrict the flow of breath but also reduce our flexibility and mobility as we move through our daily activities. The tight bras that many women wear can restrict the movements of the middle chest and back, and combined with overly tight jeans, pants, or stretch undergarments, force the breath up into the shoulders and top of the chest. The tight belts that many men wear to try to hold in their bellies keep the belly from expanding on inhalation and thus keep the diaphragm and other breathing muscles from moving as nature intended. The tight-fitting shirts and blouses that men and women often wear send a message to the nervous system to reduce the movements of the chest and back during breathing. Perhaps you remember a time when your shirt or blouse or suit jacket was so tight that you were afraid to take a deep breath lest you pop the buttons.

Another important influence on our breath is the kind of shoes that we wear. The high-heel shoes that many women wear to streamline their legs, for example, actually shape the ankles, calf muscles, thighs, and pelvis into unnatural configurations that throw the spine, belly, and diaphragm out of proper alignment and make breathing extremely inefficient. High-heel shoes and platform shoes, along with the narrow fashionable shoes that many men wear, make it virtually impossible to move in a grounded and relaxed way, which in turn tightens up all the muscles, tendons, and ligaments of the body, raises our center of gravity from our lower abdomen to our upper chest, and thus ensures a fast, tiny, restricted breath.

Self-Image and Self-Presentation

Just as important as the actual physical effects of our clothing, however, are the psychological effects. Our self-image is inevitably bound up with the particular ways we attempt to present ourselves to the world. The clothes we wear, the hairstyles we choose, the furniture in our homes, the cars we drive, and so on are all direct or indirect manifestations of this image, as advertising professionals and their clients know so well (it's how they make their living). What is not so well known is that it is possible to gain deeper access to our inner world, and thus begin to see more clearly some of the many psychological influences on our breathing, by experimenting with these outer manifestations.

Next time you go into a clothing store, for instance, ignore the clothes you are attracted to and try on some clothes that are not really "your style." Try on a whole outfit like this and look at yourself closely in the mirror. Or, on the contrary, try on clothes that you would love to wear but don't because they are too expensive. In either case, as you look in the mirror be attentive to your inner reactions to what you see. Be sure to sense your breathing. Has it changed in any way? For those of you who are really adventurous, you might try purchasing some clothes that are not "your style" and wearing them to an important social occasion.

What experiments like these show is that we are all "stuck" in a particular way of presenting ourselves not only to others but also, and perhaps more importantly, to ourselves. We are so accustomed to seeing ourselves a certain way that if we intentionally change that way even for a few minutes the various mental and emotional attitudes underlying our self-image become more visible. It is through this increased awareness that we can begin to see and release some of the internal psychological pressures on our breathing.

The Smells of Vanity

Our self-image has its smells, too, and these smells, emanating from both ourselves and others, often have a pernicious influence on how we breathe. Many years ago I worked in downtown San Francisco and spent time in offices around the entire Bay Area. I have numerous memories of getting on elevators and going into offices filled with strange, various, unpleasant mixtures of both common and exotic perfumes, colognes, aftershaves, shampoos, and deodorants. The cacophonous smells that assailed me were frequently so strong and noxious that I often had to hold my breath so as not to grimace or even gag. Or, if I didn't hold my breath, I would instinctively breathe less and breathe through my mouth so I didn't have to smell these obnoxious mixtures. At the time, I had not yet gone deeply into the various issues connected with healthy breathing, and I was little aware of my own breath. But I remember these experiences well, and I remember seeing others having the same kind of reactions.

Lest I give you the wrong idea, I do enjoy wonderful smells, especially the wind-driven smells of ocean, flowers, trees, and grass, or the subtle hint of an unusual perfume or incense. But the strong perfumes, aftershaves, deodorants, and other fragrances we often use on ourselves to cover up our own natural odors or to attract others seldom mix well, especially in enclosed environments where people come together in large numbers. In the name of spirituality and healing, some people even light candles and fill their meeting rooms with clouds of exotic incense that they believe will help transport us into higher realms of consciousness. The resulting mixture of burning candle wax and incense, perfumes, deodorants, aftershaves, and many varieties of plain old sweat, along with the exhaust fumes that one finds in large cities, often results in obnoxious smells that even the most diabolically clever among us could never have dreamed up.

The body's instinctive reaction in such situations is to breathe less, hold the breath, or breathe through the mouth to avoid the unpleasant odors. Constantly repeated over a long period of time, none of these instinctive reactions is good for our breathing.

But there's an even darker, more dangerous side to the smells of vanity. Even the best-smelling chemical fragrances can be poisonous to us. To understand why this is so, it is important to realize that the fragrance industry is not regulated. The industry is protected by trade secret law, and most of us therefore have little idea what is actually in the fragrances we use. A quick perusal of the twenty most common chemicals found in chemical fragrances makes clear that many of chemical fragrances that we use are filled with many of the same ingredients that can be found in gasoline, cigarettes, and other dangerous substances. These chemicals have been found to be associated with a variety of problems, from irritation of the trachea and lungs, to allergies, asthma, and cancer. So listen to your body when you find yourself breathing less or even holding your breath in certain places around certain smells. Get out of harm's way. And use your common sense. If you must wear a fragrance, use a natural fragrance if possible, and use it sparingly. Some people are allergic even to natural fragrances, and when people come together in enclosed spaces with little or no fresh air, the resulting smell of the various fragrances can be both unpleasant and harmful.

The Quest for the Hard, Flat Belly

Our self-image influences the way we work out, too, and thus has a powerful influence on our breath. The hard, flat belly, for instance, has become the holy grail of fitness seekers in today's society. We see it everywhere: in fashion and fitness magazines, on television, at the movies, and in fitness centers. Those of us who don't have one, want one, and those of us who do have one are sure to adorn it in tight fitting clothes that show it off to best advantage. Alas, I do not have a hard, flat belly, but if I did I would make every effort to be sure that it was capable of moving in and out during exhalation and inhalation.

At a group session with a respected physical fitness trainer that I attended a few years ago in Southern California, we were all told that we should "hold in" our bellies to support our spines as we did all the fitness exercises. We were also told to take deep breaths. Anyone with any inner ability to sense himself or herself knows quite well that it is virtually impossible to take a deep breath if your belly is pulled tightly inward. If you don't believe me, try it now. Suck your belly in and hold it there as you try to inhale deeply. But please, don't do this too forcefully as you could actually hurt yourself.

If you try this you will quickly become convinced, as indeed you should, that a strong yet soft and supple belly is needed for healthy natural breathing. Your belly needs to expand outward on inhalation so that your inner organs can move forward and down, thus allowing your diaphragm to move down farther than would otherwise be possible. It is the downward movement of the diaphragm that allows the lungs to fill more fully and efficiently. By all means, make sure your belly is strong, but hardness without softness is not strength, and developing and maintaining a hard, flat, immobile belly or overly inflexible muscles in other parts of the body, can over time, undermine your breathing and your health.[3]

Self-Importance, Vanity, and Low Self-Esteem

The self-importance, vanity, or low self-esteem often associated with our self-image has a powerful influence on our breath, and underlies much of our behavior and the way we present ourselves to the world. Have you ever watched how self-important or vain people move through the world? At their most extreme, self-important people tend to look as if they are in a state of permanent inhalation. They tend to move aggressively through the world driven by their arched spines and their almost permanently inflated, inflexible chests. Because they are so top heavy, they are generally neither centered nor grounded and often demonstrate little flexibility in their minds, hearts, and bodies.

It is also useful to notice how people with low self-esteem move through the world. At their most extreme, such people look as if they are in a state of permanent exhalation. They tend to move fearfully and hesitantly through the world led by their forward-projecting heads, which seem to pull their bent spines and their sunken chests along for the ride. Being weighed down and dispersed by the force of gravity, they struggle to regain some sense of their innate structure.

In short, with self-importance we often see a rigidly inflated chest; with insecurity and low self-esteem, we often see an overly de-flated or collapsed chest. (It is important to point out, however, that some people have learned to arch their spines and inflate their chests in military fashion in order to cover up problems with low self-esteem, so these observations don't always apply.) In both cases the diaphragm's movements are impaired, the belly, chest, and back lose their ability to expand and contract with the breath, and useable lung volume is decreased.[4] The end result is usually fast, shallow, ineffi-cient breathing.

Of course, most of us don't fit neatly into one category or the other. In fact, many of us manifest chronic symptoms of both self-importance and low self-esteem. For many years I was one of those who moved through life head first with a bent spine and a somewhat collapsed chest, vainly attempting to have my self-professed talents recognized by others. A paradoxical but lawful blend of low self-es-teem and self-importance (to cover up my insecurity) crippled my sensory awareness, tightened my breathing, and had a deleterious in-fluence on my overall health. It is only in recent years that I have begun to make conscious the previously unconscious events and emotions underlying this situation and gotten hands-on help from practitioners of Feldenkrais, Alexander, Chi Nei Tsang, and osteopa-thy to enable my posture to begin to correct itself and my breathing spaces to open more fully.

All of us, of course, experience temporary states of self-importance or insecurity in our journey through this life. This is a natural response to living and is not in itself a problem. It is only when such states become chronic in us, fueled by past traumatic events, by deep unseen emotions such as fear, anxiety, grief, and anger, and by our efforts to cover up what is really motivating us, that our self-importance or insecurity begins to dominate our self-image and to crystallize various restrictive patterns in our body, mind, and feelings. These fixed patterns, which chronically inflate, deflate, or immobilize the belly, chest, back, and spine in some manner, and which also immobilize the internal organs and tissues, make it nearly impossible to live and breathe in a full, natural, healthy way.

To truly free up our breathing in any lasting way—indeed, to free up our perception of ourselves and others and begin living more authentic lives—we need to become conscious of these patterns, as well as of the fears, traumas, and so on that feed them. We need to learn how to see our self-importance and low self-esteem for what they are—attitudinal straightjackets that distort and immobilize our perceptions, our breath, and our movement through life, and cut us off from our own life force. And we need to learn how to see and exhale the attitudes that lie at the foundation of these restrictive psychosomatic conditions.

THE POWER OF EXHALATION, OF LETTING GO

Many of us who work with our breathing, especially those of us who are attempting to explore our breathing in relation to the whole of ourselves, understand that any real, lasting transformation of the breath usually begins with learning how to exhale more completely. There are a number of anatomical and physiological reasons for this, including the obvious but often forgotten fact that if our lungs are full of stale air that has not been exhaled, there is no way we can take in the fresh air we need for optimal functioning and health.

What's more, we're clearly in trouble if our diaphragm is not strong and supple enough to help expel the old air in our lungs. Trying to inhale in such circumstances, indeed, using force to take a deep breath, as many people do in both the name of health and spirituality, will only further exacerbate the problem. Such efforts, which for most of us involve tensing our breathing muscles in some way, will further restrict our ability to inhale fully. The secret to strengthening the diaphragm lies in the exhalation. One effective way to strengthen the diaphragm, for example, is to carry out a consistent and progressive form of vocalization techniques such as toning, chanting, singing, counting out loud, and so on.

There are also important "metaphysical" reasons for beginning with exhalation. "Full exhalation and inhalation, letting go and taking in, are most possible when we are free enough to let go of the known and embrace the unknown. In full exhalation we empty ourselves—not just of excessive carbon dioxide, but also of old tensions, concepts, attitudes, expectations, and feelings. In full inhalation, which arises by itself after a full exhalation, we renew ourselves—not just with fresh air (and oxygen), but also with fresh impressions of everything in and around us."[5] When we trust in life enough to really let go, to exhale fully, inhalation occurs as a natural reflex freely and spontaneously. And when it does, it engages more of the whole of us without any effort on our part. In most cases, any effort to take in, to inhale, brings into play all the complex machinery of our self-image and its distorted functioning and simply adds more tensions and restrictions to the tensions and restrictions already present.

Our real efforts need to be applied to discovering how to be more receptive and open to the truth in our lives. Becoming more open, of course, necessitates that we find ways to see, accept, and let go of the many unnecessary fears, anxieties, expectations, assumptions, and tensions that buffer us from the reality of the present moment and that result, in large part, from the narrow, distorted ways that we view ourselves and others. When we are truly able to exhale our self-image, to become empty for a moment without a collapse of any kind, we discover a new, more authentic center of gravity and a new more creative way of living. The life force is liberated in us and brings us new, more honest perceptions and purpose, as well as inhalations and actions that are free, natural, and spontaneously appropriate to the situation at hand.

When should we practice exhaling our self-image? There really is only one time to practice, and that's right now. As the old saying goes: "Each moment is the best of all opportunities."

Practices for Exhalation and Letting Go

One of the first steps in full exhalation is to become aware of the many unnecessary physical, emotional, and mental tensions that we carry with us in almost every aspect of our lives, and to understand that these tensions derive, for the most part, from the mostly distorted, illusory image that we have of ourselves. This is no small task, since for many of us these tensions are so deeply embodied in the way we live that, if we are aware of them at all, we justify them as just a "normal" part of living. As "normal" as they might be in today's world, they are certainly not natural, and they have a powerful negative influence on our breathing, our health, and our spiritual well-being.

From the spiritual perspective, one of the inevitable results of our chronic unnecessary tension is the undermining of our relationship to "Heaven and Earth," as the Taoists would say, and to the *breath of life* that animates our being. To regain this relationship we need to consciously sense ourselves aligned properly with the earth. We not only need to allow the earth to fully support the weight of our bodies under the influence of gravity, but we also need to release the weight of our self-image, with its chronic fears, worries, judgments, assumptions, expectations, and tensions. Of course, many of us are quick to offer so-called rational reasons for carrying around all this extra psychological weight in ourselves. We have our stories ready for whoever is willing to listen. But when we look closely, we see that these reasons and stories are, in large part, our way of not having to face what is really going on in us.

As you will see in Chapter Four (in the meditative practice called Expanding Time), one of the major underpinnings of our self-image is the notion that the future is somehow more important to us than the present. For our breathing to change in any fundamental way, this attitude, of course, will also have to change. Instead of rushing into the future propelled by our identification with the momentum of our fears, anxieties, expectations, desires, and assumptions, we need to stop inwardly for a moment, feel our feet on the ground, sense our center of gravity somewhere deep in our lower abdomen, and allow our weight to be fully supported by the earth. If we can allow all four of these conditions to occur simultaneously, the tight grip of our self-image on our breathing will begin to relax; our mind and nervous system will quiet down; our tense, chronically raised shoulders will drop without our chest collapsing; our compressed or bent spine will begin to straighten and lengthen both upward and downward; our exhalation will slow down and become more complete; and our inhalation will begin to fill and animate more parts of ourselves.

Of course, there are many techniques to slow down the exhalation and make it more complete, and I have included some of these in this book. But lest these techniques merely bolster a distorted or illusory self-image that already has us under its sway, we often need to explore the work of exhaling and letting go without any techniques at all. We often need to remember to listen within for the call of our own essential being, of our own essence, and to let go of what stands in the way of hearing this call—our identification with or attachment to the habitual associative thoughts and emotions that arise from and support our self-image. These automatic ego-based thoughts and emotions may never truly vanish, but we don't need to believe and lose ourselves in them. We don't need to feed them with our inner attention and life force.

We can and should, of course, practice letting go any time we can remember to do so, but the practice of listening within for the call of our own essential being is sometimes more possible in the morning when we first awaken and at night just before falling asleep. It is at these special times, which metaphysically speaking represent birth and death, that we can sometimes hear both the boundless silence of our own inner being and the boundless energy of breath and life as it manifests through us—without the fixations, expectations, and manipulations of our self-image. It is at these special times that we can, as the Taoists say, truly learn to "exhale the old and inhale the new." It is at these special times that we can experience the embrace of the "metaphysical breath," a breath that goes beyond the physical and opens us to an expansive sense of our own extraordinary wholeness.

The Shoulders and Feet Exercise

Here is a simple practice that can help you see your self-image in action more often, and give you an opportunity to let go of it in the moment. The practice will also greatly benefit your breathing. Try it as often as you can throughout the day.

Phase One: The main effort is to remember to keep your shoulders down and relaxed in the ordinary activities and circumstances of your day, whether these activities and circumstances are stressful or not. When you suddenly catch yourself with tense or raised shoulders, notice what you are identified with[6] at that moment and immediately sense your breathing to see where it is taking place in your body. What mental, emotional, or other psychological weight are you carrying? What unnecessary tensions can you feel? As soon as you have a clear sensation of what is going on, let your shoulders drop down and simultaneously let these tensions dissolve downward through your body into the earth.

Phase Two: After you have tried this exercise with your shoulders for several days, you can include the following practice. After you have observed your shoulders, your breathing, and any tensions, sense your feet touching the floor or the earth and let them relax.

Have the sensation that your feet are spreading out on and into the ground, and that the relaxation of your feet is attracting your tensions downward. If you are standing see if you can sense your entire weight being supported by the ground or floor. If you are sitting on a chair, see if you can sense your entire weight being supported by both the chair and the ground beneath your feet. Sensing your weight in this way will allow gravity to lengthen your spine and release the tensions in your belly, chest, and back. Notice how this influences your breathing, helping it, without any effort on your part, to become freer and fuller, engaging more of your belly, back, and chest in an effortless way. Notice also how you are more present to what is going on at that moment and how some things that may have been bothering you seem suddenly to be seen from a new, less-troublesome perspective.

Phase Three: Try the exercise walking slowly for fifteen minutes or more every day in a park, your garden, or down the street. The key is to take your time, really sensing your shoulders and feet and letting them relax as you walk. Be sure to smell the air and sense its warmth or coolness as it goes all the way into your lungs. Listen to everything taking place in and around you as you consciously let go of your identification with your habitual thoughts and feelings, as well as the concerns and preoccupations that they represent. Notice how your breathing changes as you enter more deeply into the present moment.

You can also try the Conscious Walking Practice in Appendix A.

Lengthening Your Exhalation and Revitalizing Your Lungs

This exercise, which I first learned in the Taoist tradition as part of the Six Healing Sounds or Exhalations, is said by the Taoists to be useful for problems such as colds, coughs, and congestion, and to help transform the energy of grief and sadness into the energy of courage. It is also used by various breathing therapists and teachers to help lengthen and strengthen the exhalation and stimulate full, free inhalation. It is a great exercise for anyone who wants to breathe in a more complete and natural way—who understands that authentic breathing is not something that we do but rather something that we allow—the action of being breathed from the inside.

Either sitting or standing in an upright position, inhale gently and naturally through your nose. Then exhale only through your mouth while making the sibilant s sound (ssssss), the sound of hissing, the sound of a radiator as steam is released from it. Continue making the sound until you sense that you have about 10 percent of your exhalation left, finish exhaling slowly through your nose, and wait for the inhalation to arise by itself (be sure to inhale only through your nose).

While exhaling with the s sound, do so slowly and evenly, listening carefully to the sound. See if you can keep the sound very steady, of equal intensity through the entire exhalation, without using excessive effort. The first time you try the exercise, try it every other breath. Try it one time while exhaling with the sound and sensing how the inhalation arises by itself. Then exhale naturally through your nose, let the inhalation arise by itself, and exhale with the sound again.

Once you can hear that the sound is steady and even, you can try the exercise several times in a row without alternating. When you are comfortable with the exercise, you can add the following inner work. As you make the sound on the out-breath, use the power of your intention to exhale whatever thoughts, emotions, or attitudes seem to be buffering you at that moment from yourself. You can try this exercise for up to five minutes at a time several times a day.

Taking Off Your Self-Identity

Breathing practices by themselves can bring many benefits, but they need to be supported by fundamental changes in our inner attitudes. To learn how to let go, to exhale ourselves, we need to practice in many ways. Here is a practice that you can try when you go to bed at night and arise in the morning, and that you can learn to integrate into your daily life.[7]

As you take off your clothes to get into bed, have the sense that you are taking off your self-identity, your past, and your anticipated future, and that you are entering gladly and voluntarily into the unknown. Take off your thoughts, emotions, worries, and so on. Get into bed naked both psychologically and physically (if you wish to wear something, put on something that you have not worn during the day). As you lie in bed ready for sleep, there is no past or future; there is only the full sensation of yourself now as a breathing being.

When you wake up in the morning, don't just jump out of bed mechanically driven by everything that you believe you have to do. Before opening your eyes and getting out of bed, let yourself return for a minute or two to this unknown sensation of yourself as a breathing being alive right now. Listen, sense, and feel. Perhaps you can hear the question: "Who am I?" arising from deep within.

Four

Going Deeper — Practices and Meditations for Self-Exploration

OVERVIEW

The question "Who am I?" is the most honest, far-reaching question we can ask ourselves, the question which puts us directly in front of the mystery and miracle of both our breath and our existence. Yet from childhood on we are given superficial answers to this question, answers that denude the question of its power to awaken us — answers that take the unknown out of our lives. Or worse, we are told that it is not even a question worth asking.

In this collection of six practices and meditations, you will have an opportunity to see how your breathing can help you go deeper into an exploration of the unknown, of who you really are. You will have an opportunity to make a relationship not only with the physical parts of yourself of which you are usually unaware, such as your inner organs, but also with deeper levels of consciousness.

Conscious Breathing offers a powerful first step for discovering your own natural, authentic breath and for experiencing the intimate relationship of your breathing to every aspect of your life. This step has to do with learning how to listen within to the subtle movements and energies of your life force.

The Six Healing Exhalations, based on ancient Taoist principles, will help you make contact with your internal organs. The practice will not only help you learn how to regulate your organs and balance your emotions to some extent but will also, as a byproduct, help your breathing by improving the functioning of your diaphragm.

The Smiling Breath offers a simple yet powerful method for sensing and relaxing some of your internal tensions and attitudes and beginning to experience a sense of ease and spaciousness both in your internal organs and in your life.

Expanding Time offers an antidote to the speeding up of time that is taking place in our stress-filled world and shows you how your breath can help you expand your sense of the present moment.

The Breath of the Heart will help you open up your breathing and experience a profound, heart-felt appreciation for the miracle of your life. It is through this appreciation for our life as it is that we can begin to experience a sense of the boundless.

The Boundless Breath will support your quest to go beyond the confines of your habitual self-image, your sense of *I*, and begin to experience your own underlying, boundless nature.

CONSCIOUS BREATHING

As we discussed earlier in the book, the foundation of all self-directed, meditative work with breathing is conscious breathing, or breath awareness. By learning to listen to our breath, to follow the movements of our breath consciously in ourselves without any kind of manipulation, we can begin to move toward the unknown in ourselves—toward real freedom. To follow our breath requires that we become quiet inside, that we learn to be present to ourselves without any judgment or analysis. It requires that we give up our sense of knowing ourselves, and reside instead in pure sensing and receptivity. As we explore in this way, we will experience new dimensions in ourselves and learn in depth about the relationship of breathing to our physical, emotional, mental, and spiritual lives.

Sit now on a chair or a cushion. (To practice while standing, stand in the posture described in A Conscious Standing Practice in Appendix A.) Unless you have a back injury of some kind, it is better not to use the back of the chair for support. Your spine should be relaxed but erect. Close your eyes, and simply sense yourself sitting. Rock forward and backward gently on your sit bones until you find a relative sense of ease and balance while sitting. Don't slump backward onto your tailbone (coccyx). This area is filled with nerves and is one of the body's key energy centers. Slumping back on this area will have a deleterious influence on both your awareness and your health. If your spine starts tightening up anytime during the practice, simply rock forward and backward or side to side gently on your sit bones to help relax your spine and back.

Sense Your Entire Body

Once you've found a comfortable yet erect sitting posture, let your thoughts and feelings quiet down. Have the sensation that they're settling downward into your body, like tea leaves in a cup of tea. One very effective way to support this "inner quieting" is by becoming interested in the overall sensation of your body. Start by allowing impressions of your weight to enter your awareness. Really let yourself sense your entire weight on the chair, floor, or ground.

Once you can sense your weight clearly, include as much of the sensation of your skin as possible. When you can feel the tingling, the vibration, of your skin, then sense your overall form, the outer structure of your body, including any tensions in this structure. Sense yourself sitting there, letting your kinesthetic and organic awareness become increasingly alive. As your inner sensitivity increases, you will begin to experience your sensation as a kind of substance or energy through which you can receive direct impressions of both your inner and outer life.

Include Your Breath

Now that your inner attention has stabilized somewhat and become a bit stronger, include your breath in your awareness. Follow your breath—not with your thoughts but with your inner, organic ability to sense and feel. Sense any movements or sensations associated with your breath anywhere in your body. Let yourself really sense these movements of inhalation and exhalation, expansion and contraction, as well as their limitations and restrictions, in the context of the whole sensation of your body. Notice how being aware of your breathing influences your sensation of yourself. Don't try to change anything. Work in this way for at least ten minutes.

Following Your Breath in Stages inside Your Body

Now you're going to follow your breath deeper inside your body. Be aware of your breath as you inhale and exhale. Sense the temperature and vibration of the air as it flows from the tip of your nose into and out of your nasal passages on inhalation and exhalation. Take several breaths focusing only on the sensation of the air going into and out of your nose.

Now continue to sense the temperature and vibration of the air as it flows into and out of not only your nose but also your throat on inhalation and exhalation. After several breaths, sense the air flowing all the way from the tip of your nose down through the bottom of your trachea. After several more breaths, sense the temperature and vibration of the air as it flows into your nose, through your throat and trachea, and all the way down into your lungs on inhalation, and back out on exhalation.

When practicing in this way, be sure to take several gentle breaths during each stage, and don't move on to the next stage until you can clearly sense the temperature and vibration of the air. Let the air touching these various tissues help your nose, throat, trachea, and lungs relax. The more relaxed these areas become, the freer your breath will be and the more expansive your sense of yourself will become. Above all, do not manipulate your breath in any way during this practice. If you catch yourself starting to think or dream, just acknowledge this and bring your attention back to following your breath in the context of the whole sensation of your body.

Subtle Currents of Breath Energy

As you become quieter inside, you may notice subtle vibrations, subtle currents of breath energy, moving up and down and through your body on inhalation and exhalation, and these energies may arouse entirely new sensations and feelings of yourself. Just take note of the existence of these sensations and feelings and continue following the movements of your breath without any effort to analyze or interpret what is happening. Allow your breath, especially on inhalation, to draw your awareness deep inside your body.

After you've worked in this way for fifteen minutes or so, rub your hands together until they are warm and put them one on top of the other on your navel area. Sense how your belly immediately becomes more involved in your breathing. Sense how it opens on inhalation and closes on exhalation. You may feel a vibration beginning to develop deep inside your belly, as though some kind of special energy is collecting there. When you can experience it clearly, let the vibration spread everywhere, refreshing all the cells of your brain and body.

When you're about ready to stop, let go of any effort to direct your attention, and take a couple of minutes to enjoy the entire energetic sensation of yourself sitting there, alive, breathing, thinking, feeling, sensing. Notice how you are now more present, more consciously alive, to the whole of yourself.

Conscious Breathing During Your Daily Activities

When you're finished, simply get up and move on into the activities of your day. During these activities, however, check in with yourself every couple of hours and sense your breathing. Just observe and sense. Don't try to change your breathing in any way. Include your emotions, thoughts, postures, movements, activities, and so on in your awareness. Notice whether your breathing is slow and relaxed or fast and tense. Notice whether your breath is smooth and comfortable or choppy and uncomfortable. Notice whether you are holding your breath or it is flowing freely and easily. Sense where your breath seems to originate. Notice whatever you can without analysis or judgment. Simply be present to yourself and your breath for a minute or so at a time in the midst of whatever you are doing.

Include Your Thoughts and Emotions in Your Awareness

Over time, as you continue practicing daily in this way, and as your sensation of yourself becomes finer, more sensitive, and more expansive, you will begin to observe your thoughts and emotions as they start to take form—but before they absorb your complete attention. Let them come and go as they wish, but do not occupy yourself with them, analyze them, or judge them in any way. As they come and go, just include them in your awareness as part of the reality of the moment. If you are able to include them in your awareness without analysis or judgment, you will receive increasingly global impressions of the subtle relationships that exist between your thoughts, emotions, postures, sensations, energy, and breath. It is through this multilayered work with awareness that the habitual boundaries in your breath, thoughts, feelings, tensions, and so on can begin to dissolve.

THE SIX HEALING EXHALATIONS

The Six Healing Exhalations is an ancient Taoist breathing practice that uses the power of special sounds on exhalation to help contact and heal the organs of the body and transform the so-called negative emotions associated with these organs into the so-called positive ones. I first learned a version of this practice during a workshop with Taoist master Mantak Chia, who calls it "The Six Healing Sounds,"[1] and have since come across various versions of it in the Taoist canon. It is important to realize that from the Taoist perspective it's not a matter of ridding ourselves of negative emotions and having only positive ones, but rather of making sure that our emotions are in balance and that our internal organs do not become overstressed or overheated. The Taoists believe that unbalanced emotions and overstressed organs disrupt our energy flow and create numerous restrictions in how we perceive and live.

Description of the Sounds

The six sounds are related to the major organ systems of the body and their associated energy channels. They are also related to specific colors. You can use both the sounds and the colors in this practice.

Lungs and Colon: The first sound, sssssss, the sound of hissing, acts on the lungs and colon, and is related to the nose. The sound is said to be useful for physical problems such as colds, coughs, and congestion, and to help transform the energy of grief and sadness into the energy of courage. The color associated with this sound is white.

Kidneys and Bladder: The second sound, WHOOO, the sound you make when you blow out a candle, acts on the kidneys and bladder, and is associated with the ears. This sound is said to be useful for increasing your overall vital energy and for problems such as cold feet, dizziness, and lack of sexual energy, and to help transform the energy of fear into the energy of gentleness. The color associated with this sound is dark blue.

Liver and Gall Bladder: The third sound, SHHHH, the sound that you use when you want someone to be quiet, acts on the liver and gall bladder and is associated with the eyes. This sound is said to be useful for eye problems, anorexia, and vertigo, and to help transform the energies of anger or jealousy into the energy of kindness. The color associated with this sound is green.

Heart and Small Intestine: The fourth sound, HAWWWW (as in the word "hawk"), acts on the heart and small intestine and is associated with the tongue. It is said to be useful for heart disease, insomnia, ulcerations of the tongue, and night sweats, and to help transform the energies of hatred, arrogance, or impatience into the energy of love, compassion, or patience. The color associated with this sound is red.

Spleen, Stomach, and Pancreas: The fifth sound, WHOOOO (guttural, in the back of the throat), acts on the spleen, stomach, and pancreas and is associated with the mouth. It is said to be useful for digestive problems, mouth ulcerations, muscle atrophy, and menstrual disorders, and to help transform the energy of worry or anxiety into the energy of fairness or balance. The color associated with this sound is a golden yellow.

Triple Warmer: The sixth sound, HEEEEE (hissed through the teeth), acts on the triple warmer, which is more or less equivalent to the three breathing spaces (from the feet to the navel, from the navel to the top of the diaphragm, and from the top of the diaphragm to the top of the head). There is no particular emotion associated with this sound. It is said to be effective for sore throats, abdominal distention, and insomnia and is also used to help harmonize the overall energy flow of the body. There is no color associated with this sound.

Practicing the Six Healing Exhalations

To ensure the overall health of all the organs and the harmonious movement of energy throughout the body, the Six Healing Exhalations or Sounds should be practiced daily in the order given above. Each sound should be repeated at least three times, inhaling through the nose and exhaling very slowly through the mouth as you make the sound. If you have a particular problem associated with a specific organ or emotion, you can spend more time with the associated sound, repeating it as many times as you like. Be sure to rest for several breaths when you change from one sound to the next.

You can also use these sounds, as we have already done with the lung sound, to help lengthen your exhalation and increase the coordination, strength, and elasticity of your diaphragm and other breathing muscles. The lung sound and the liver sound are particularly useful for this aim.

Inhale Pure Energy; Exhale Toxins

The practice itself is extremely simple. You can undertake it in any posture. Whichever organ you are working with, sense that you are inhaling fresh, pure energy directly into that organ and that the entire area is opening and expanding. As you exhale using the associated sound, simultaneously sense any toxins or excess heat in the organ being carried out of your body with your exhalation and that the entire area is closing or contracting. If you enjoy visualization, you can inhale the color associated with each sound, and exhale with the sound visualizing a dark, cloudy, or gray color leaving your body with your breath. Another approach is to sense that you are inhaling the unknown into yourself and exhaling the known.

To help get in touch with your various organs (fig. 4.1), you should rub your hands together until they are very warm and, depending on the sound you are about to make, put them on your body over the area of the primary organ you are working with, and keep them there as you inhale and exhale. Use your attention to sense the entire area in and around the organ. Work with the organs in the following order: *lungs* (right hand on your chest over your right lung on the right front part of your rib cage and your left hand over

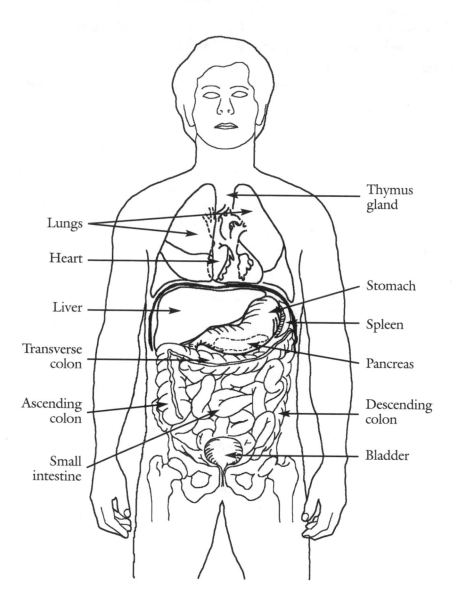

Lungs

Heart

Liver

Transverse
colon

Ascending
colon

Small
intestine

Thymus
gland

Stomach

Spleen

Pancreas

Descending
colon

Bladder

FIGURE 4.1
Internal organs

your left lung on the left front part of your rib cage), *kidneys* (palms on your middle back with your middle fingers touching), *liver* (lower right front portion of your rib cage), *heart* (slightly to the left of the center of your chest), and *spleen/stomach* (the left lower front portion of your rib cage).

For the last sound, the triple warmer sound, as you inhale raise your hands just above the top of your head (palms facing downward and fingers pointing toward one another if you're sitting or standing, and palms facing toward the opposite wall if you're lying down on your back). If you are sitting, stretch your legs out as far as you can in front of you with your feet flat on the floor. If you are lying down, lie down on your back with your legs comfortably extended.

As you exhale using the sound, move your hands slowly down your body with the intention to help dispel any toxins or excess heat from your body. As your hands reach hip level, turn them so that your palms are facing your body and your fingers are pointed toward your toes and continue the movement of your hands until your arms and hands are fully extended as you complete the exhalation. Have the sense that toxins and heat are leaving your body through your fingertips and toes.

With any of the sounds, in addition to exhaling audibly, you can also experiment with exhaling inaudibly, concentrating the vibration of the sound inside the organ. If you are with people, you can dispense with the use of your hands and simply make the sounds inaudibly to yourself. Make sure, however, that you use your inner awareness to sense the primary organ associated with each sound.

The Six Healing Exhalations can be practiced safely at any time of the day or night, but as a healing practice it is particularly useful when you first get up in the morning or just before going to bed. If you must eat before doing the practice, wait for at least thirty minutes before beginning. When you're finished working with the entire series, be sure to spend a couple of minutes just sensing any changes that have taken place in your breathing, as well as in your overall sensation and feeling of yourself.

THE SMILING BREATH

A genuine smile has great power not only to relax and benefit others, but also to bring about deep levels of relaxation in the person who is smiling.[2] This is especially true in today's high-pressured world, where tense, frowning faces are the norm.

The Smiling Breath,[3] which is an adaptation of a meditation from the Taoist tradition, brings together the power of the smile with the power of the breath in an integrated practice for health, healing, relaxation, and wholeness. It involves becoming aware of the specific emotions, both negative and positive, traditionally associated with the various internal organs. The key is to allow your emotions to come into the full light of your inner awareness without trying to do something about them. Be sure to give yourself plenty of time to sense and feel what is taking place within as you work with this meditation.

To begin, sit quietly either on a chair or a cushion with your eyes closed. You can also do the practice in a standing posture (see A Conscious Standing Practice in Appendix A) if you are able to stand for at least twenty minutes. If you sit, your hands should be palm down on your knees or folded gently together on your lap. If you stand, be sure that your feet are parallel about shoulder-width apart, your knees are slightly bent, your shoulders are relaxed and down, and your arms are hanging easily at your sides, palms facing back. Let your feet relax into the floor or ground. Feel how the earth is supporting you.

After a couple of minutes simply sitting or standing like this, sense your whole body simultaneously, including any tensions and emotions. Let these tensions and emotions begin to flow or settle downward, like impurities in a glass of water. Don't stir them up by thinking about them or making an occupation out of them. Sit or stand for at least five minutes in this way.

Now include your breathing in your overall sensation of yourself. See if you can sense the various movements of breath in your body—from your lower belly (or even your feet) all the way up to your head. Be careful, however, not to force your breath in any way. Allow your exhalations and inhalations to proceed on their own.

Sensing and Relaxing Your Eyes

Staying in touch with the movements of your breathing, begin to sense your closed eyes. Gently rotate, or spiral, them several times in every direction you can. Then stop and let them relax back into their sockets. Your eyes are linked to the autonomic nervous system, which controls and regulates the action of your glands and organs. By relaxing your eyes you can help relax your entire body and nervous system.

Let the Sensation of Relaxation Spread into Your Face

Once you feel that your eyes are relaxed, let the sensation of this relaxation spread through your whole face, even into your tongue, ears, and the bones of your skull and jaw. Stick out your tongue and stretch and spiral it in many different directions. Let it relax inside your mouth. The relaxation of your face, and especially your tongue, will help free you from the incessant inner talking that contributes to so much unnecessary tension and stress.

Now visualize with your eyes closed someone you care about smiling at you. Let their smile enter you. Smile back at them. Sense how your eyes and face relax even more. If you are unable to conjure up an image that makes you smile, then simply smile intentionally. Relax your eyes even more, turn up the corners of your mouth, raise your cheeks, and do the best you can in "putting on a smile." If you can maintain this effort for several minutes, you will soon find yourself smiling quite genuinely and effortlessly.

Sense Your Breath Being Touched by the Smile on Your Face

Make sure that you're still in touch with the various movements of your breath. Each time you inhale, sense the air entering not only through your nose, but also through your face and eyes. Sense your breath being touched by the smile on your face. Watch how the smile transforms your breath. It's as though the smile makes your breath even more vibrant and expansive.

Breathe into Your Thymus Gland

Now you're going to direct your smile inwardly toward yourself, guiding your smiling breath into your major organs as shown in figure 4.1. As you breathe through the smile on your face, let your smiling breath flow downward, like water, through your jaw and neck and into your thymus gland behind the upper half of your sternum (breastbone). The thymus gland is an important part of your immune system. Sense the thymus gland opening and closing on the in-breath and the out-breath.

Breathe into Your Heart

Now, sense the area of your heart. Rub your hands together until they are warm and put them over your heart. Let the warmth from your hands penetrate deep inside your heart. Can you begin to sense your heartbeat? Check to make sure you are still smiling, and then direct the smiling breath down into this deepening sensation of your heart. Have the idea that you are breathing through your heart. See if you can sense your heart actually relaxing as you smile and breathe through it. See if you can sense your diaphragm touching and massaging your heart as you exhale. Do you feel any hatred, arrogance, or impatience in your heart? Can you also feel a sense of appreciation for simply being alive?

Breathe into Your Lungs

Now let the deep, relaxed sensation of your heart spread to the sides into your lungs. Direct the smiling breath into your lungs on both sides of your heart. Can you sense the muscles of your chest becoming more supple and relaxed as you breathe into and out of your lungs? Can you sense your lungs expanding and contracting more completely inside your chest? Do not use force—only sensation. Can you feel any grief that you may have? Can you also feel the courage to be yourself?

Breathe into Your Liver

From your lungs, let your sensation expand into your liver on the lower right side of the front of your rib cage. Smile and breathe into this area. Sense the area around the liver expanding and contracting gently and releasing any unnecessary tension. Can you sense your diaphragm massaging your liver as you inhale? Can you feel any anger you may have toward yourself or others? Can you also feel a sense of kindness and compassion?

Breathe into Your Stomach, Pancreas, and Spleen

Check to be sure that you still have a smile on your face. Then let your sensation expand into your stomach, pancreas, and spleen on the lower left side of the front of your rib cage, and watch how your smiling breath follows your sensation into those organs. See how the tissues around these organs begin to soften as you breathe into and out of your stomach. Can you feel any worries that you may have? Can you also feel a sense of balance and fairness?

Breathe into Your Kidneys

Now allow the sensation to move into your kidneys and the adrenal glands that sit on top of them, in the lower and middle back area on both sides of your spine. See how your smiling breath moves into your kidneys. Notice how your back and kidneys expand and contract a bit as you breathe into and out of your kidneys. Sense any unnecessary tensions in and around your kidneys being released. Can you feel any fear you may have? Can you also feel a sense of gentleness?

Breathe into Your Bladder and Sexual Organs

Now let your smiling breath follow your sensation into your bladder and sexual organs. As you breathe into and out of this area, you may sense your whole lower abdomen opening and filling with energy. You may also begin to have a new sense of your own internal power.

Collect and Absorb the Energy

Now, as you inhale, sense your abdomen expanding with the spaciousness of your smiling breath. Sense the warmth and energy in your abdomen. As you exhale, do so slowly through your mouth as though you were gently blowing out a candle. Keep most of your attention in your abdomen and allow the comfortable, spacious sensation that you have there to spread simultaneously into all your organs, tissues, and bones.

Once you feel that your awareness of this process is strong enough, you can add the following dimension to this practice. As you exhale, sense the *smiling energy* being absorbed into your organs at the same time that you sense any inner tensions or toxins leaving with the exhalation. As you gain proficiency in this practice, you will discover that it has enormous power to energize you and support your well-being.

Smile Often into Your Heart

You should practice the full Smiling Breath meditation daily for at least fifteen to twenty minutes at a time. Throughout the day, however, you may catch yourself getting lost in anger, fear, anxiety, worry, and other negative emotions. When this happens, take an inner snapshot of the precise configuration of your body, thoughts, and emotions at that moment. Then bring your attention to your heart and sense the entire area, letting it relax. Smile and breathe into and through your heart for at least one minute, allowing yourself to appreciate the great gift of being alive now and here.

Practice the Smiling Breath in Your Daily Life

As you undertake the Smiling Breath, check frequently to be sure that you still have a smile on your face. After several weeks of practice in quiet circumstances, you will be able to bring about many of the same results with just the slightest sensation of an inner smile. This will enable you to practice in the midst of the pressures, stresses, and conflicts of your everyday life. It is in these conditions that you will see how this practice can help you see and transform your habitual emotional reactions and inner attitudes and liberate your breathing.

THE BREATH OF THE HEART

The expression "The Breath of the Heart" is not just a beautiful and evocative metaphor. It also conveys a way of breathing that is as boundless as are the heartfelt feelings of love, compassion, and appreciation. When we are able to breathe with spacious inhalations and long, full exhalations, our diaphragm actually uplifts and massages our hearts.

As we have already discussed, however, most of us do not exhale fully and with ease. In this practice, you are going to experience how breathing through your heart can release some of the restrictions in the armor of your self-image and allow you to make deeper connections with yourself and others.

Listening to Your Tensions and Your Breath

The first step in this practice is to experience consciously how you actually breathe now. You need to observe with full sincerity how the unnecessary tensions in your body and mind restrict not only your breath but also your feeling of life. This work of listening to your breath is not just a matter of hours, or days, or weeks, or months, but is rather a lifetime work. For our breath always echoes these tensions and the way in which they clamp down on us, undermining our health, depriving us of the sensation of inner and outer spaciousness, and suffocating us in the process.

As you experience the coming and going of these unnecessary tensions in the various conditions of your life, you will soon discover that they are intimately bound up with your negative emotions—especially anger, fear, worry, and anxiety—many of which repeat endlessly, as well as the thoughts that support them. By following your inhalation inward in the midst of these tensions and emotions, you will discover that it creates, if only for a moment, a bit more space and openness. Through the sensation of this momentary opening, something in you can relax and enable you to come into a new, more direct resonance with yourself. The experienced spaciousness of your in-breath will help call forth deep reservoirs of space within the tissues, energies, and vibrations of yourself. As you exhale, you will then be able to feel and let go of these restrictive thoughts, attitudes, and emotions.

The Need to Engage Our Hearts

For this process to go deeper, however, the heart must take part. For it is through the heart, and especially through feelings such as love, compassion, and appreciation, that we can truly open to receive and embrace life. We need only remember times when such feelings were present in our hearts to realize the way in which they opened us to ourselves and others. We know that it is only through a more open heart that we can find a real sense of spaciousness in our lives.

How can we intentionally engage the heart in our breath? What practices can we undertake? There are many approaches to this, coming from many of the world's spiritual traditions. One approach, for example, has to do with inhaling into oneself the pain and suffering in the world and then exhaling love and compassion. Though an ongoing practice such as this can have powerful results, many of us might find it difficult to undertake such a practice in a genuine way. But you are certainly welcome to try it.

Sensing and Feeling Your Heart

Another approach, which may be more accessible to many of us, has to do with learning to sense and feel our hearts more often throughout the day. You can undertake this practice in a classic meditation posture. You can also try it whenever you remember in the other circumstances of your life. You can even try it right now as you read these words.

The first step in the practice is to sense your weight being supported by the earth. Whether you are sitting, standing, walking, lying down, or whatever, sense the actual interface between your body and the earth. If you are standing, for example, focus your attention on the sensation of your feet on the floor or ground. If you are sitting on a chair, focus your attention on the sensation of your buttocks (especially your sit bones) touching the chair and your feet touching the floor. Put all your attention on these sensations until you begin to feel that you are being fully supported by the earth itself.

Now feel and sense the entire area of your heart. You can support this process by putting one or both hands on your chest over your heart and sensing the warmth and energy coming from your hands.

Smile into your heart. Allow any tensions in the area, anything that feels frozen or contracted, to simply dissolve from the warmth of your attention, your hands, and your smile. Feel how your breath begins to expand and to be drawn into your heart. Sense the gentle breeze of your breath moving through and softening your heart with each inhalation and exhalation.

Appreciating the Miracle of Being

As you continue to sense yourself being supported by the earth and your breath engaging your heart, you may begin to experience feelings of love and appreciation. Though you can, if you wish, try to re-experience past moments of feelings such as these, you will see that it is possible to come directly to a deep and immediate sense of appreciation for your life, with everything (both positive and negative) that it includes, at this very moment. As you inhale and exhale intentionally through your heart, see if you can feel the great miracle of being that your life as it is represents—the fact that you are alive now and here, in a vast universe that no one really comprehends. As you continue working quietly in this way, you may inexplicably find yourself breathing within a boundless space of presence radiating inward and outward from your heart, a space in which the present moment— *now*—takes on an entirely new significance.

But beware! If you approach this practice as merely another exercise, you will never experience the fullness that it can bring. More than any technique, what is really needed is a deep effort of listening anew, of being open to the unfathomable miracle of ourselves as breathing beings. It is through this openness, this spaciousness, that we can go beyond our little selves and touch what is true in ourselves and our lives.

EXPANDING TIME

A serious exploration of breathing and breath takes us into many realms, including chemistry, physiology, psychology, and even metaphysics. As we have seen, the way we breathe reveals a great deal about the way we live—including our thoughts, feelings, perceptions, and relationships with ourselves and others. When we work seriously with our breath, we are, whether we know it or not, bringing about changes, or at least the possibility for changes, in many other areas of our lives. One of the biggest changes we may begin to experience is in our relationship to time.

The Speeding Up of Time

One of the most profound and least understood aspects of breath is its relationship to time. As citizens of the twentieth and twenty-first centuries, most of us find that time seems to be speeding up. This speeding up of time is associated with increasing levels of stress, and stems mainly from our perception, from the increasingly complex way we see, feel, and sense our lives. In our daily lives we are called upon to deal with rapid shifts in our attention, thoughts, feelings, and actions as a result of a barrage of ever-changing tasks, demands, information, fears, worries, and so on. This constant shifting of our attention and the corresponding demand this places on our brain and nervous system causes many of us to live in a low-grade but chronic fight or flight or freeze state, in which unnecessary tension robs us of our vital energy, and the constant release of hormones such as adrenaline and cortisol undermines our immune system and throws us into increasingly negative states of disharmony.

Because the nervous system is so adaptable and resets its internal thermostat to function at this higher frequency of activity, we end up taking our chronic states of anxiety, impatience, worry, and fear for granted, assuming that they are somehow "normal." Instead of going directly to the root of the problem, to the limiting, self-defeating ways that we perceive the world, we try to do things to create more time for ourselves—such as purchasing the latest, fastest, and most powerful computers, or rushing forward toward time to get some place or accomplish something faster. One sees people (and ourselves), for example, at bus stops, in lines, at stop signs, walking down the street, and so on impatiently waiting or rushing as though future time were somehow more important than *now*. And this rush away from *now* into some imagined future seems never to stop. Even on our vacations what we're planning to do next often seems to be more important than what we're actually doing.

Unfortunately, this ubiquitous attitude, along with all the things we often do to try to save time, usually makes time appear to move and disappear even faster. It's not time that needs saving—it's us. Our time seems more and more filled with things that from the perspective of real harmony and happiness are either counterproductive or meaningless.

"Time Is Breath"

G. I. Gurdjieff said that "time is breath."[4] And J. B. Priestly once described our time-starved situation as that of a knight who gets on his horse to go in search of time, not realizing that "time is the horse he is riding." If time is indeed breath, and it is also the horse we are riding, then perhaps we can look toward our breath to discover a new, more conscious relationship to time in our lives.

For anyone who cares to look, it is certainly clear that the growing stress, anxiety, worry, and disharmony that many of us experience in this period of human history is closely associated with the fast, shallow upper-chest breathing that many of us experience in our daily lives, even when we are at rest. Such breathing is not just the result of chemical or mechanical imbalances in our body, but also stems from our increasing sensation and feeling of not having enough time and space in our lives. And this sensation comes in large part from our brain and nervous system, which is often in a state of emotional alarm. The truth is, as adaptable as we are as human beings, we are not designed for the kinds of chronically high-speed stressful lives that many of us live, and we pay a heavy price for it in terms of both our health and our happiness.

The Full Expanse of the Present Moment

If time is indeed breath, however, then there is an intelligent and healthy way out of this dilemma. The secret is in discovering a new inner attitude that can help us slow down our breathing and live in the full expanse and freedom of the present moment. Looking toward the future for some change in our lives without learning how to fully experience "the horse we are actually riding" is doomed to failure. Pushing ourselves into the future, as many of us do under the influence of our latest high-speed information technologies, undermines the rhythms and wisdom of the human organism and suffocates our breath and our life.

To open ourselves to our own inherent rhythms and wisdom, we must learn to experience through direct awareness the terrible effects that our time-conditioned life has on our health, well-being, and perception, and we must learn to open the breathing spaces of the body and find our own unconditioned breath—a breath that will most certainly reveal itself as longer and slower than our usual breath, which is now held captive to the stress-producing emotions of fear, anger, anxiety, and worry.

What is needed to help bring this about is not just work with breathing (though this is certainly necessary), but also a radical change of perception—the conscious, heartfelt experience of love, kindness, nonjudgment, and compassion, both toward ourselves and others. These feelings, which act as antidotes to the poisonous time-eating emotions that many of us experience day in and day out, can help harmonize our nervous system and bring our attention into the miracle of the present moment. They represent the felt appreciation for what exists here and now both in ourselves and others.

There is a simple practice that you can undertake to support this change in perception. It has two phases: quiet work by yourself and work in stressful circumstances.

Phase One: Practice Conscious Breathing

Sit or stand quietly each morning and practice Conscious Breathing for at least fifteen minutes. Then, as you sit or stand, sense the area around your heart. Feel how the area starts getting warm and your tensions in the area begin to dissolve, like ice turning into water. When the area of your heart feels more relaxed, on the inhalation say silently and slowly to yourself "alive." On the exhalation say silently and slowly to yourself "now." Feel these words resonate in your heart as you begin to sense and appreciate your own alive-ness. See if you can be aware of the whole phrase "alive . . . now," from beginning to end as you inhale and exhale through your heart. See if you can experience your breath, "alive . . . now," as the present and only moment of your life. Let both your exhalation and your inhalation slow down and lengthen as your awareness of the present moment begins to expand and deepen. Notice the natural rest—the pause—at the end of the exhalation. During this pause, let your awareness expand to include the whole sensation of yourself. Notice any feelings that arise, but don't try to interpret or analyze them.

After at least ten minutes of working in this way, let go of any effort and simply enjoy the feelings, sensations, and impressions that have arisen. Appreciate your own "being-ness," your own aliveness. Notice how the present moment seems to have expanded, and how there seems to be more time and space for you to simply unfold and be.

Phase Two: Practice in the Middle of Stressful Situations

After you have tried this for a week or two quietly on your own, try this work with your heart when you are in the middle of your daily activities, especially when you are in the midst of a stressful situation of some kind. Remember, "time is breath" and "time is the horse you are riding," so it takes no extra time to do this meditation in action. Just sense your heart and inhale and exhale "alive . . . now" through your heart as you deal with the situation in front of you. You will be surprised at how the heartfelt appreciation of your own existence now can shield you from and transform many of the stress-related problems in your life and begin to expand your experience not only of time, but also, perhaps more importantly, of yourself.

THE BOUNDLESS BREATH

Those of us who are called to an honest exploration of ourselves have no choice but to include the metaphysical dimensions of the breath, the relationship of breath to spirit and to the unknown. It is though our breath that we can begin to experience the unknown without going anywhere other than where we are right now.

As we have already discussed, learning to let go, to exhale completely, is in fact a movement into the unknown. When we truly let go, we do not know what will happen next or where we will find ourselves. In letting go, we give up, if only for a moment, a sense of controlling our lives. And even though we know in our heart of hearts that such giving up of control is vital not only for our breath, but also for our inner growth and our happiness, many of us are afraid of allowing it to happen.

Here I would like to propose a special meditative practice in which you will use your breath as a pathway into the unknown dimensions of yourself. The regular practice of this meditation can help create a new harmony between your three centers of perception—your head, heart, and body. It can also help you go beyond these centers toward an entirely new sensation of your inner being, your unconditioned, boundless nature.

Sit Quietly

Begin by sitting quietly toward the front of a firm chair. Make sure that your spine is upright yet supple. Close your eyes, and fold your hands together in your lap or put them palm down over your knees. Rock gently forward and backward on your sit bones until you find a comfortable yet erect posture. Check your feet to be sure they are relaxed and flat on the floor. Just sit quietly for a few minutes, doing nothing except sensing and smiling into yourself. Let the inner quiet, the silence, begin to grow and to envelop whatever thoughts, feelings, and sensations are taking place.

Ask "Who Am I?" with Your Head

Now, focus your attention on your head. Have the sense that you are breathing into and out of your head. After a couple of minutes of breathing in this way, ask yourself with your head "Who am I?" Don't allow yourself to be seduced by any particular answer. Simply ask the question and, listening from the silence, observe, and let go of any "answers" or other thoughts that appear. Ponder this question in this way for at least five minutes.

Let Your Tension Dissolve Downward

Direct your inner attention again to the very top of your head. Let the sensation of the top of your head soften and come to life, releasing any stress or tension you may feel there. Then let this sensation of softening, of dissolving, gradually move downward through your head, your ears, your face, your mouth, your neck, and so on through your whole body and down into and even below your feet. Do not hurry this process. Simply sense how your stress and tension are releasing downward through your entire body and finally into the ground beneath you.[5]

Ask "Who am I?" with Your Heart

Now, putting your hands on your heart, breathe gently into and out of your heart and ask "Who am I?" again, but this time, see if you can actually feel the question resonating from and in your heart. Work in this way for at least five minutes.

Sense the Whole of Your Body

When you're ready, let the whole sensation of your body enter your awareness, including the movements of your breath. Follow your breath as it moves from the tip of your nose, through your nasal passages, into your throat and trachea, and down into your lungs. Sense how the tissues of your body seem to open as you inhale and close as you exhale in a deep, natural rhythm. Don't try to do anything. Just follow, sense, and watch. Observe any thoughts or feelings that take place, but don't make an occupation out of them. Continue to follow your breathing like this for at least five more minutes.

Now put your hands on your belly and sense how your belly expands or wants to expand as you inhale and retracts or wants to retract as you exhale. Don't use force. Just sense your belly opening and closing (or wanting to open and close) with each breath.

Now breathe into and out of your entire body and ask "Who am I?" again, this time with your sensation. Let the question come alive and vibrate in every cell of your body for at least five minutes.

Notice the Pause at the End of Your Out-Breath

Now let go of any intention with regard to the question "Who am I?" and notice the natural pause in your breathing cycle at the end of the exhalation. Include this pause in your overall awareness of yourself. The great mystical traditions have spoken of this space between

exhalation and inhalation as an entryway into our unconditioned nature, into our underlying unbounded reality as pure consciousness.
It is in this space between our out-breath and our in-breath, a silent
spaciousness that is always there beneath our thoughts, feelings, and
sensations that we can more readily begin to let go of everything we
think we know about ourselves and open ourselves to the unknown.
It is in this space that we can begin to experience the transformative
power of the living question "Who am I?"

Continue to follow your breathing, paying special attention to the
space between your out-breath and your in-breath. With each breath,
allow this space to become a kind of sacred resting ground, a place
where you can, if even for only a moment, safely give up your self-
image, your self-identity, and experience your own real nature. It is
here that you can return home. Don't try to *do* anything. Just sense
and feel.

As your outer breath continues, and as this space begins to manifest itself as pure consciousness, let yourself become one with it. See
how your thoughts, sensations, feelings, and breath are all somehow
contained within this consciousness. Feel the miracle of yourself here
and now, consciously alive in the boundless ocean of the unknown.

When You're Ready to Finish

When you're almost ready to finish, let go of any experiences you
may have just had and come back for two or three minutes to the
whole sensation of your body and the movement of your breath
from the tip of your nose down into your lungs. Then let go of following your breath and just be present for a few moments to the sensation of yourself sitting there. Finally, let go of the special sensation
you have of yourself. It will come to you again, unexpectedly, but
don't try to keep it or force it. Now smile to the ever-present miracle
and mystery of yourself, gradually open your eyes, and, when you are
ready, return to your so-called ordinary life.

Other Core Teachings and Practices

THE TEN SECRETS OF AUTHENTIC BREATHING

1. If possible in your daily life, inhale and exhale only through your nose, even when you are doing aerobic exercise.
2. Sense the movement of your breath frequently in the midst of your everyday activities. Remember not to hold your breath.
3. Be sure your belly stays relaxed. Let it expand as you inhale and retract as you exhale. Touch it and massage it frequently. Your belly is the foundation of your breath.
4. Breath is life and movement. Let your breath engage and fill every part of your body, especially your belly, back, spine, and chest.
5. To transform your breathing, start with your exhalation, with "letting go."
6. A long, slow exhalation helps harmonize your diaphragm and turns on your "relaxation response."
7. Sense the natural pause after exhalation; let yourself rest there for a moment.

8. Let your inhalation arise by itself, when it's ready.
9. Sense the various breathing spaces of your body several times a day. Smile into these spaces and observe how your awareness helps them open and close effortlessly.
10. Remember, you are a breathing being, alive right now and here. Let yourself feel the mystery and the miracle of your breath and your life as often as you can.

THE IMPORTANCE OF BREATHING THROUGH YOUR NOSE

It is extremely important to learn to breathe through your nose except when you are doing special breathing exercises that call for mouth breathing, or when you are unable to breath through your nose because of injury or illness.

Basic Principles

When we breathe through our nose, the hairs that line our nostrils filter out particles of dust and dirt that can be injurious to our lungs. If too many particles accumulate on the membranes of the nose, we automatically secrete mucus to trap them or sneeze to expel them. The mucous membranes of our septum, which divides the nose into two cavities, further prepare the air for our lungs by warming and humidifying it.

Another very important reason for breathing through the nose has to do with maintaining the correct balance of oxygen and carbon dioxide in our blood. When we breathe through our mouths we usually inhale and exhale air quickly in large volumes. This often leads to chronic hyperventilation (breathing excessively fast or breathing too much air too quickly for the actual conditions in which we find ourselves).

It is important to recognize that it is the amount of carbon dioxide in our blood that generally regulates our breathing. Research has shown that if we release carbon dioxide too quickly, the arteries and vessels carrying blood to our cells constrict and the oxygen in our blood is unable to reach the cells in sufficient quantity. This includes the carotid arteries, which carry blood (and oxygen) to the brain. The red blood cells also become "sticky" and are slow to release the oxygen into the cells. The lack of sufficient oxygen going to the cells of the brain can turn on our sympathetic nervous system, our "fight or flight" response, and make us tense, anxious, irritable, and depressed. There are some researchers, such as Dr. Konstantin Pavlovich Buteyko, who believe that mouth breathing and the associated chronic hyperventilation that it often engenders can contribute to the onset of asthma, high blood pressure, heart disease, and many other medical problems.

There's one more good reason for nose breathing. In his book *Dr. Fulford's Touch of Life*, famed osteopath Robert C. Fulford, D.O., has this to say: "Remember: always try to breathe through your nostrils, and not through your mouth, because air must contact the olfactory nerves to stimulate your brain and put it into its natural rhythm. If you don't breathe through your nose, in a sense you're only half alive."

Nose-Breathing Difficulties

If it is difficult for you to breathe through your nose, it could well be the result of allergies or of a structural problem of some kind, for example a problem with your septum. A broken nose at any time in your life could easily cause such a problem. In such cases, it may be necessary for you to see a medical specialist.

Difficulty breathing through your nose could also be the result of what and how much you eat. Habitually eating too many calories or too many of the wrong kinds of foods, especially sugar and high-glycemic carbohydrates (these kinds of carbohydrates, which are quickly converted into blood sugar, include flour, white rice, cold cereals, pasta, bananas, and so on), can cause your insulin levels to surge in order to reduce blood sugar levels. According to Dr. Barry Sears, "Elevated levels of insulin promote the overproduction of bronchoconstrictors."[1] Bronchoconstrictors narrow our airways and thus make it more difficult to breathe and to take in sufficient oxygen. Anyone who has had an asthma attack knows what having too many bronchoconstrictors feels like.

Difficulty breathing through your nose could also just be the result of habitual mouth breathing. As I have discussed elsewhere in this book, the more you breathe through your mouth, the more carbon dioxide you will lose, which can cause the tissues in your nose and other airways to swell and become congested and thus make it more difficult to breathe.

Nose Breathing for Aerobics and Sports

Many people who breathe through their noses in their everyday lives believe that it is normal to breathe through their mouths when working out. But some physical therapists, breathing therapists, athletic trainers, and health care professionals point out that this is a mistake.

Peg (Meg) Jordan, a registered nurse and founder of *American Fitness Magazine*, is one of them. In her book *The Fitness Instinct,* she recounts the story of John Douillard, D.C., an Ayurvedic practitioner who worked with tennis stars like Martina Navratilova. Douillard had to convince them to bring their workout "intensity down to a level where they could breathe through their noses." Though they resisted this at first, Douillard was able to convince them through a battery of sports tests that training in this way "actually improved their performance, stamina, focus, and coordination." Jordan writes: "Douillard knew that breathing through the mouth tends to inflate only the upper lobes of the lungs, which are connected to sympathetic nerve fibers, the branch of the nervous system that activates the flight-or-flight fear response. . . . When you switch to nose breathing, you inflate the entire lung, including the lower lobes, which are connected to the parasympathetic branch of the nervous system, the branch that calms the body, slows the heart rate, relaxes, and soothes. Through proper nose breathing, you employ both branches of the nervous system. At times the foot is on the brake; at times, it is on the gas. The back-and-forth fluctuation is a balancing act that your body intrinsically knows how to do and that your mind appreciates."[2]

In other words, proper nose breathing brings a balance to our nervous system that mouth breathing cannot bring. Once we have accustomed ourselves to working out in this way—doing only as much as we can do while still breathing through our nose—this balance ensures the most efficient, effective, and satisfying use of our physical, emotional, and mental resources.

Nasal Dilators

There are some people these days who promote the use of nasal dilators to help people take in more oxygen through the nose. Recent research, however, seems to show that whereas nasal dilators do seem to help people who have breathing problems during sleep, they boost neither oxygen intake nor athletic performance for people during waking hours.[3]

This should come as no surprise to those who have explored their breathing to any depth. For people with normal lung function, getting sufficient air into and out of the lungs is only the first step. It is equally important for the oxygen in the lungs to be efficiently transported into the blood and from the blood into the cells of the body and brain. Inhaling and exhaling more air in a shorter period of time (which nasal dilators make possible by decreasing airflow resistance) may facilitate the first step, but it can, through excessive loss of carbon dioxide, actually reduce the amount of oxygen available to the body and brain.[4] What's more, airflow resistance itself is an important aspect of the entire breathing process, and any changes in this resistance can have often unforeseen consequences. It is clearly not just a matter of the quantity of air that we breathe into the lungs, but also of whether or not the way we breathe, eat, and live facilitates the efficient transport of oxygen where it is needed in our brain and body.

THE ART OF EFFORTLESS EFFORT IN DOING BREATHING EXERCISES

Without knowing it, many of us who work with our breathing actually try too hard. Our efforts are based on force, on will power, not on skill and sensitivity. Instead of working with the laws of natural, healthy breathing we work against them. The more we *try* to breathe naturally, the more tension we create in our minds, emotions, and bodies, and the more we restrict the movement of our diaphragm and other breathing muscles. This not only wastes energy, but it also floods the body with excessive adrenaline and metabolic waste. Unnecessary tension increases our heart and breath rates. Unnecessary tension also causes our sensory system to go on alert, sending distress signals to the brain, which further increases our level of stress and tension.

One of the main keys to learning natural, healthy breathing is a sense of effortlessness and comfort. As you work with the Belly Breathing exercise, for instance, be sure to work slowly, gently, and patiently. When you put your hands on your belly, be sure that your hands are warm. Really let yourself feel the warm, comforting sensation of your hands on your belly. This will help you relax and will attract the movement of your breath into this part of your body.

As you work comfortably in this way, you will begin to work more from the sensation of what is actually happening rather than from a picture of what you think should be happening. This is important. It is through increasing sensitivity to our inner sensations that we can begin to make great strides in our work with breath.

Using the Belly Breathing exercise again as an example, you may sense that your belly wants to expand as you inhale, but that something keeps it from this expansion. When you sense this, there will be a temptation to use your muscles to push out your belly. Resist this temptation. Simply stay with whatever sensation you have there, and gently massage all around your navel, gradually widening the area of your massage to include your entire belly. As you continue this gentle massage, the muscles in your belly will gradually begin to relax. Let yourself enjoy this sensation of relaxation, and you will soon find your belly more involved in your breath. If you practice working in this way, eventually you won't have to use your hands at all. Simply putting your attention inside your belly will be enough to attract your breath there.

To sum up: as you practice the exercises in this book, be sure to try less and enjoy more. The key is effortless effort. For most of us, our efforts are filled with unnecessary muscular contractions and tensions. When our body is freed from these unnecessary contractions and tensions, it knows how to breathe in the most appropriate way possible in any situation.

A CONSCIOUS STANDING PRACTICE

As human beings, we spend most of our time in three basic postures: lying down, sitting, and standing. These postures represent different ways of being in the world. Lying down, which releases us from the major influences of gravity on our bodies, activates our parasympathetic nervous system, a sense of our vegetative reality. It is a posture that generally relaxes us and leads to unconsciousness and dreams. Standing, which maximizes the influence of gravity on our bodies, activates our sympathetic nervous system, a sense of the aims and aspirations related to our self-image. It is a posture that lends itself to alertness and action. Sitting, which is a kind of middle ground, activates both our parasympathetic and sympathetic nervous systems, but to a lesser degree than either lying down or standing.

It is a posture that naturally lends itself to meditation and calm reflection.

Though most meditative techniques are taught in sitting postures, the recent influx into the West from China of qigong standing practices has opened the door to a powerful new (in the West) approach to self-study and self-transformation. Authentic qigong standing practices (qigong simply means energy work) are designed to help conserve, balance, and transform our inner energies, as well as to help open us to the energies of the earth, of nature, and of the heavens. Because these practices are able to help harmonize all of the various energies available to us, they are ideally suited to healing and self-transformation.

Learning to Let Go

One of the most powerful influences of qigong standing, however, one that is sometimes overlooked, is its ability to help us learn how to "let go" at both the physical and psychological levels. You may have heard about or seen taiji or other masters who, while standing in a totally relaxed posture, cannot be moved from their position or lifted off the floor, no matter how small they are or how big the person attempting to push them or lift them. This has to do with learning how to release any unnecessary tension in our bodies and to allow our weight to settle downward through our bones, tendons, and ligaments into the earth. Such a person is supported by the earth not just physically but also energetically. One does not have to be a master to learn this, although one usually does need the help of a teacher to demonstrate the principles involved in such standing.

If one works with this practice both deeply enough and long enough, one begins to understand that letting go physically is not possible without letting go psychologically, and that letting go psychologically is not possible without letting go physically. One sees with absolute certainty that the old, stale ideas, attitudes, emotions, and impressions of our mind are equivalent to the unnecessary tensions and habits of our bodies, and that they are irrevocably linked. Body and mind must be worked on simultaneously if any real transformation is to take place. Before we can undertake such a transformation, however, we need to see that this linkage is indeed a reality in our lives. As an experiment, over the next several days observe as often as you can how you actually stand in the various conditions of your life. Wait until you've had a chance to experiment in this way before continuing on with this practice.

We Seldom Just Stand

If you are honest in your observations, you will see that, in fact, you seldom "just stand," that you almost always do something else as well. You will catch yourself automatically and unconsciously leaning against walls, crossing your hands over your belly or chest, putting your hands in your pockets, twisting your body in some way, shifting your weight back and forth, and so on. As you observe yourself in these various standing postures, see if you can sense your breathing and the various tensions in your body. See if you can also notice the kinds of thoughts and feelings you are having. Try this for a few days before reading further.

Once you've received clear impressions of the ways that you normally stand, try a new experiment. When you stand, whether you're with people or alone, allow your weight to sink equally onto both feet and let your hands simply hang at your sides, palms facing behind you. Be sure that your weight is sinking to the middle of your feet, not to the balls of your feet or your heels. Have the sense that the earth is supporting you, and that there is nothing that you need to do except to sense yourself standing in this way. Try carrying on a conversation with someone this way. As the conversation continues, can you continue to stand in such a way that your weight is evenly balanced and that you maintain a sense of openness and vulnerability? See if you can notice the precise moment when the openness vanishes, when you twist, turn, lean, shift, or use your hands to cover or protect some part of your body. If you try this experiment seriously over a number of days or weeks, you will receive many new, informative impressions of yourself.

Now you're ready to take the experiment a bit further. By yourself, try all the same things standing with your feet parallel to each other, about shoulder-width (or less) apart, with your knees just slightly bent. Relax your shoulders, shoulder blades, and chest. Gently adjust your coccyx (your tailbone) so that it is more or less pointed directly down toward the ground. When this happens, the arch in your lower back will naturally flatten out. See if you can sense your lower back and sacrum connecting directly to your legs. (Remember to let your arms hang naturally at your sides with your palms facing back.)

Once you are more or less comfortable in this posture (fig. A.1), use your attention to slowly scan your entire body from the top of your head to the bottom of your feet, noting where there is any unnecessary tension in your tissues and muscles. As you scan your body, do not attempt to change anything. Simply observe and sense. Above all, keep breathing; don't hold your breath.

Once you reach the bottom of your feet, start again from the top of your head, and see if you can gradually release any unnecessary tension in your tissues and muscles downward through your body into the earth. As you try this, you will begin to sense a new dimension of inner balance, a sense of being supported by and rooted to the earth. It's as though your breath comes up through your feet from the earth itself. Start out by standing this way for at least five minutes a day. Once your legs and pelvis begin to feel comfortable in this posture you can move on to ten or fifteen minutes a day or more.

After undertaking this practice for a couple of weeks, begin to experiment with it in your ordinary life—talking to friends, waiting in line, and so on. The idea is not to take the same exact posture that you take when working alone, but rather to have the continuing sen-

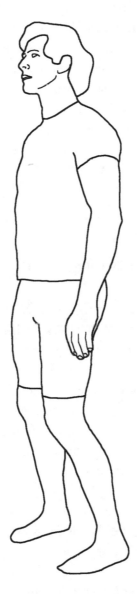

FIGURE A.1
Basic standing position

sation of releasing all your muscular tension downward through your body into the earth. See if you can "just stand," with your weight equally distributed through both feet and your arms at your sides, totally open to whatever impressions or perceptions the moment may bring. If you observe a thought or emotion making some part of your body tense, just return to the sensation of releasing this tension downward into the earth. As you continue to work in this way in whatever circumstances you may find yourself, you will begin to discover a deep sense of relaxation not just physically, but also mentally and emotionally. You will find yourself spontaneously "letting go" of much that is unnecessary both at that moment and in your life.

A CONSCIOUS WALKING PRACTICE

Though we generally take it for granted, walking can be one of the most profound activities of our lives. As human beings, we walk for many reasons: to get some place, to stay fit, to relax, to explore, to enjoy, to get away, to ponder, or some combination of these and many other motives. Sometimes we walk for no other reason than it seems like the right thing to do. Though the virtues of walking are immediately apparent to most of us, we seldom consider the act itself—about *how* to walk in order to gain the most enjoyment and benefit from this remarkable activity.

When I ask people how they walk, most of them are puzzled by the question. They believe that however they do it, it gets the job done—it gets them where they want to go or increases their cardiovascular fitness. From the standpoint of goals such as these, it may not matter exactly how we walk, as long as we walk quickly enough. But from the standpoint of our breathing and overall health and well-being, it matters greatly. The rigid, automaton-like movement that many people call walking often does more harm than good, both physically and psychologically.

Walking is a vital activity not only for our bodies but also for our spirits. In addition to giving our cardiovascular system some of the exercise it needs, walking can also help relax us, energize us, and reduce the stress of our everyday lives. It can open us to the deep interrelationships and fluid rhythms of movement and breath, and help intensify our awareness of our rich, inner world of sensation. It can help produce the chemical substances that give us a sense of vitality and well-being. To fully experience the benefits of walking, however, one needs to approach it not as an activity we already know how to perform, but rather as an art we need to learn.

Learning the Art of Walking

The first step in the art of walking is awareness or mindfulness—the awareness of how you actually walk now. Be careful here that you do not equate mindfulness with thinking. If you do, you'll suffer the fate of the centipede that became paralyzed and could not move when someone asked it which leg it moved first when it started moving.

Next time you walk take a few minutes to put your attention on yourself. How do you feel as you walk? What is your real motive for walking? Are you in a hurry to get it over with, or are you experiencing and enjoying each step and breath of air you take? If you're anxious or impatient, chances are that you'll have a lot of unnecessary tension in your muscles. And this will bring discomfort and quick exhaustion. The art of conscious walking depends on the rhythmical and harmonious movement of all the parts of your body without unnecessary tension.

Opening and Closing the Joints of Your Body

As you continue to observe yourself, sense the various parts of your body that move as you walk. Observe the range of these movements. For example, do your arms swing comfortably and naturally forward and backward, in opposition to your feet, helping to open and close the joints and breathing spaces of your body, or are they held back by tension in your shoulders and neck or by some mental "image" you have of what you're supposed to do with your arms? In this regard, neuroscientist Candace Pert tells us that when she walks, she lets the "opposite hand swing forward with each step. . . . Somehow this sets left brain-right brain information flowing, breaking up old patterns of worry and rumination. I've found that it's impossible to stay stuck in unproductive old thought patterns when I move my body this way."[5]

In the same vein, does your pelvis remain rigid as you walk or does it swing naturally from side to side? Allowing your pelvis to swing naturally as you walk will help open and close your joints; support the movement of blood and lymph throughout your body; exercise all your internal tendons, ligaments, and muscles; create waves of movement that will massage your spine and inner organs; and open up your breathing spaces.

Becoming Aware of Your Feet

Now put your attention on your feet. Can you sense each foot at the moment it touches the ground? Can you sense each foot when it leaves the ground? Do your feet feel tight? Relaxed? How do they move in relation to the ground? Do they come down gently or hard? Do they come down flat, on the heel, or on the ball? Do they roll from heel to toe? (If they come down hard on your heels, for example, you may eventually injure your spine.) Can you feel your toes? Play with the way your feet touch the ground. See if you can discover a gentle rolling motion, in conjunction with the swinging motion of your arms and pelvis. If you can, any unnecessary tension in your feet, legs, pelvis, and shoulders will relax, and you will feel yourself simultaneously grounded and extremely light. You will experience gravity as a force that not only gives you weight but also lifts you and propels you forward effortlessly step by step.

Sense Your Breathing

Now see if you can sense your breathing. Sense each inhalation and exhalation as it takes place. Where in your body does your breath seem to begin—in your feet, your belly, your chest, your throat? The Taoist sage Chuang Tzu said that true human beings breathe with their heels, while the majority of us breathe with our throats. As you begin to release unnecessary tension in the way that you walk, you will discover your breathing reaching deeper down in your body, bringing parts of yourself to life that you seldom sense. As this occurs, the efficiency and capacity of your respiratory system will increase. This will make it possible for you to walk longer with less fatigue. And, perhaps even more important, you will sense your body in a new, more complete and energetic way.

Walking inside the Energy Atmosphere of Your Breath

Now try this powerful practice. As you walk, have the sense that you are walking inside the energy atmosphere of your breath. You can support and enliven this experience by being attentive to the expansive sensation of your body as a whole, the atmosphere that surrounds and interacts with your body as you walk, and the subtle movements and energies of your breath as you inhale air from and exhale air into this atmosphere. As you walk, have the sense that there is really nowhere to go except deeper inside the energy atmosphere of your breath—your life force.

The Art of Walking Begins with Awareness

As we said before, the art of walking begins with awareness, as everything real in our lives does. To be mindful while walking is an extraordinary experience, and it can have some of the same benefits that doing taiji or qigong with full awareness can have. Mindful walking supports our health and increases our sense of well-being. It helps us to experience life directly as it moves us and moves through us. It helps us perceive our inner and outer worlds with greater clarity. Each step is a new adventure, another opportunity to uncover new aspects of ourselves and the world in our journey through space and time. Each step is an opportunity to return home to ourselves and to experience the miracle of our own existence now and here, wherever we may be in our boundless journey through space and time.

APPENDIX B

Helpful Breath-Related Exercises for Daily Living

A SAFE, SIMPLE EXERCISE FOR STRESS RELIEF

Excessive stress is involved in a wide variety of medical conditions, including heart disease, high blood pressure, ulcers, acid reflux disease, strokes, and many other illnesses. Though most of us have heard that deep breathing can help us relax in the midst of stressful situations, many of us do not really know how to breathe deeply. We do not know how to quiet our minds and emotions and release the unnecessary tension in our diaphragm, ribs, belly, and back that restricts our breathing. As a result, our efforts to deal with stress through deep breathing often result in shallow, fast breathing which tends to make us even more nervous, anxious, and tense than we already are.[1]

Though it is extremely important to your breath and health to learn how to quiet your mind and emotions and to release unnecessary tension in your breathing muscles, there is a simple breathing practice that you can use in the meantime to help you relax. In this approach, you simply emphasize and lengthen your exhalation. The long exhalation helps turn on your parasympathetic nervous system, your "relaxation response."

Using this technique, there's nothing to do except to make sure that your exhalation is longer than your inhalation. You don't have to count to do this. Just put your attention on your breathing as you exhale. Sense the air from your lungs going out slowly and gently through your nose. When you're finished exhaling, don't put your attention on the inhalation. In fact, don't make any kind of effort to inhale at all. Just wait for your inhalation to arise by itself. Take several complete breaths in this way.

If, after several breaths, your exhalation still isn't longer than your inhalation, simply imagine that you are gently blowing out a single candle as you exhale slowly and effortlessly through pursed lips. Take several more breaths in this way, and you will soon find yourself beginning to relax. To deepen this relaxation, you can hum for several breaths.

This is an extremely safe exercise, so you can practice it as often as you like. The key is to breathe gently and effortlessly.

SLOWING DOWN YOUR BREATHING

Though physiology textbooks tell us that the average breath rate for adults at rest is about twelve to fifteen breaths a minute, serious practitioners of qigong, yoga, taiji, and so on generally breathe at a much slower rate than this. And research from various quarters has shown that slower breathing generally brings with it many physical, emotional, and mental benefits.

In a study published by L. Bernardi et al., in the May 2, 1998 issue of *The Lancet*, for example, researchers working with cardiac patients at the University of Pavia, Italy, established an optimum healthy breath rate of six breaths a minute. When you consider that the average resting breath rate is twelve to fifteen times a minute, this represents a substantial reduction in breath rate. Patients who learned to slow down their breathing through special deep-breathing exercises apparently ended up with higher levels of blood oxygen and were able to perform better on exercise tests. According to the report, low blood oxygen, which is common in cardiac patients, "may impair skeletal muscle and metabolic function, and lead to muscle atrophy and exercise intolerance." The authors of the study concluded that their findings support other research "that report beneficial effects of training respiratory muscles and decreasing respiratory work in (cardiac heart failure patients), or physical training in general."

It is important to realize that the world's great spiritual traditions employ various ritual methods, most of which have the effect of slowing down the breath without making any special effort to do so: meditation, mantras, prayer, chant, qigong, taiji, and yoga.[2] Many of us, however, do not participate in such activities, and so, unless we undertake special breathing practices, our breath and our life are usually at the mercy of whatever high-speed individual or cultural stresses we face.

There are numerous safe ways to slow down your breathing, the most important of which is to learn how to breathe with the help of all your breathing spaces. Over time, the practices in this book will help bring this about. In the meantime, there are some safe, natural methods that you can practice for several minutes each day on a regular basis that will help slow down your breathing. By training for several minutes each day for several weeks, you may well find your breath spontaneously slowing down at other times of the day as well.

Here are two simple and effective sound-supported breathing practices that you can use to lengthen your exhalation and slow down your breathing to about six breaths a minute. The aim of these practices is to provide an easy way to make each complete breath (inhalation/exhalation/pause) last about ten seconds each. The following practices will not only help bring this about, but will also begin to train your diaphragm to move farther through its complete range of motion in a free and natural way.

The Timed Counting Practice

To prepare for this practice you will need a watch or clock with a second hand. The first step is to calculate your average inhalation/exhalation at rest (sitting). The simplest way to do this is count the number of complete breaths that occur in one minute. Then simply divide that number into sixty seconds. If you are like most people, the resulting number will be in the range of four to five seconds for a complete breath (inhalation/exhalation/pause). When timing your breath, do not make any special effort, and do not try to breathe more or less or faster or slower. Just breathe the way you usually do.

Once you have an idea of the length of your usual breath, the next step is to intentionally lengthen your exhalation (not your inhalation) so that each complete breath takes about ten seconds. Here is the way you will do this. Start timing your breath with your inhalation; then as you exhale simply count quickly and evenly in a quiet voice from one to ten. Count two or three times to ten without a pause and then simply let the rest of the air out through your mouth (as though you were gently blowing out a candle) and wait for the next inhalation to arise by itself. If each breath (from the beginning of one inhalation to the next) takes about ten seconds or more, great. If not, simply add another set of counting from one to ten as you exhale.

Once you have fine-tuned this process (which should only take a few minutes), and have really sensed what it feels like to breathe at a rate of about six breaths a minute, you will not need to look at a clock again for awhile. As you try this exercise over a period of days and weeks, however, you should check yourself every once in while, since you may find your inhalation lengthening and deepening a bit by itself, and you will need to adjust your exhalation appropriately. If you naturally find yourself breathing fewer than six breaths a minute at rest—that's fine. Just be sure that your exhalation is as long or longer than your inhalation.

Try this exercise for at least ten minutes on a daily basis. After practicing for several weeks, you will probably begin to notice your breath rate slowing down by itself even when you're not trying the exercise. When doing the exercise, be sure to inhale through your nose and exhale through your mouth as you count in a quiet whisper. When you're not doing this or other special exercises, it is best to breathe entirely through your nose if possible and let your breath flow naturally.

The LA LA LA *Practice*

Another simple practice you can try to extend your exhalation—with or without any effort to time your breath—is to repeatedly and rapidly sing (or silently vocalize if you are with other people) the sound LA . . . LA . . . LA . . . LA during exhalation. Follow the same basic instructions that are given in The Humming Breath practice in Chapter One in the section on Sound-Supported Breathing. As described there, be sure to discontinue the sound before you run completely out of air, finish the exhalation slowly and quietly through your nose, and wait for the inhalation to take place spontaneously by itself. This is a wonderful practice to do on a daily basis. Like the counting practice above, it will help your diaphragm move freely and easily through its full range of motion, thus helping to squeeze your lungs and massage all your internal organs, including your heart. It will also help you relax.

BREATHING TO TRANSFORM ANGER

Chronic anger has become an integral part of our stress-filled modern world. People today vent their anger almost anywhere they can—spreading negativity and disharmony everywhere. We're so accustomed to expressing our anger in an angry way that not only does it feel quite natural, but we also often feel self-righteous about doing so. As I pointed out in my book *The Tao of Natural Breathing*, however, some researchers have found that, depending on how we do it, expressing our anger can be dangerous to our health. Those of us who experience frequent anger often find ourselves dwelling incessantly on it and justifying it inwardly or else expressing it outwardly, often in strong emotional outbursts. However vital and important it might seem at the moment, the end result of expressing our anger either internally or externally is often a racing heartbeat, the undermining of our immune system, increased blood pressure, and a depletion of energy.

It is possible, however, to begin to free ourselves from our anger and to lessen its impact on us through a combination of special awareness and breathing practices. The next time you notice that you're angry, for instance, instead of dwelling on it inwardly, expressing it outwardly, or trying to suppress it, simply listen to your anger as it manifests at that moment throughout your body. Sense how it feels. Notice the posture you're in and any tensions or constrictions in your breathing. Take a deep impression, a kind of internal snapshot, of what your anger is doing to your body, as well as of the underlying thoughts and feelings that are fueling the anger. This can all be done instantaneously, in a moment of inner sincerity and awareness.

Then, without trying to hide from what you are experiencing, simply count (mentally) at a steady pace the length of your inhalation and then the length of your exhalation. Then, for your next seven breaths, inhale to the same count but double the count of the exhalation. So, for example, if you found that your inhalation lasted four counts and your exhalation three, count to four for your next seven breaths as you inhale, and to six as you exhale. (You can actually dispense entirely with the counting if you like. The key to this exercise is simply to lengthen your exhalation. This will help turn on your parasympathetic nervous system—your "relaxation response.") After breathing in this way for seven breaths, take another deep impression of yourself. Include your body, emotions, and breathing. See how your need to express your anger either to yourself or others has changed. Are you still as angry as you were?

It's important when trying this exercise to remember that you will have a tendency to say to yourself "I'm too angry to do this exercise right now." Or you might say, "But I've got to say something to this person right now. I can't just let them get away with this." Or you might even say, "It's unhealthy not to express my anger." If you hear yourself making such statements to yourself when you are angry, take a moment to look at yourself both from deep inside and as if from the outside. If you can really experience yourself more objectively at that moment you will sense what your anger is doing to you, and you will want to try the exercise immediately.

We need to find the courage to face our anger with full consciousness, express it responsibly when necessary, and transform its energy into something that is useful to us. If you persist in trying the exercise at the very moment you sense that you are angry, you will soon find yourself being able to give up expressing it, or able to express it in a less mechanical, more helpful way. You will also find that you have more energy for whatever needs to be done. What's more, as you become more and more aware of your breathing, you will start perceiving your anger earlier, before it reaches the point of no return. This will enable you to deal with it in an intelligent, responsible way.

BREATHING TO REDUCE PAIN

The way we breathe can have a powerful influence on the way we experience pain. Deep breathing, for example, can often reduce the intensity of the pain we are feeling. One of the reasons that deep breathing can be so effective in pain reduction is that the lungs have a large concentration of peptides, the "partial proteins that are involved in thought and feeling," and these peptides communicate with the PAG, the periaqueductal gray area located in the midbrain. This area of the brain contains many receptor sites for the natural opiates that the body produces. Deep breathing, along with other kinds of alterations in our breathing, can influence "the profile of pulmonary peptides," help communicate with the PAG in the mid-brain, and thus increase the opiates in the body. The end result is a change in our pain threshold.[3]

Many of the practices in this book will, of course, help to slow down and deepen your breath. One excellent practice for this pur-pose is the Belly Breathing practice, in the touch-supported breath-ing section of Chapter One. In addition, the following exercise can be effective in helping to reduce or even eliminate pain. If you are not certain of the cause of the pain, however, be sure to check with your doctor before attempting to reduce or eliminate it. This exer-cise can also be used to reduce stress, and may be useful for those with asthma, emphysema, and other chronic breathing problems.

Next time you're experiencing pain or stress, just put a smile on your face. Though it will feel unnatural at the beginning, it will soon feel natural if you can hold it for at least a couple of minutes. Once you are smiling, have the sense that you're directing your smile in-wardly into your whole body. Then, as you inhale, sense yourself in-haling not just through your nose but also through the smile on your face. Let the energy of the smile combine with the energy of your breath, and direct this energy down into the area that hurts or that is tense and contracted. As you exhale, do so through pursed but relaxed lips (as though you are gently blowing on a single candle without actually blowing it out), and feel that you're releasing any pain, discomfort, or tension with the exhalation. As you inhale, allow your abdomen to expand outward. As you exhale, allow your abdomen to gently contract inward. This will help deepen your breath.

Be sure that the exhalation takes longer than the inhalation. This will help you relax. Work like this for a minimum of five minutes at a time. The key is to be gentle. Don't try to force anything. If you do, you'll just increase your pain or stress. This is a very safe exercise that you can try any time of the day or night.

RELAXING YOUR FACE MUSCLES FOR FREER, EASIER BREATHING AND MORE ENERGY

Those of you whose work requires extreme visual concentration (and the list of occupations requiring such work is a long one, especially in this age of computer technology) can improve your work and increase your energy by making sure that your face muscles are relaxed and by looking away frequently from the work you are doing. This will help you breathe in a freer and easier way.

Here is how it works. When your face muscles become tense and your eyes become fixed on anything too long, diaphragmatic movement decreases. This makes your breathing shallower and less efficient. What's more, this shallow breathing decreases the lymph flow in your body thus reducing the effectiveness of your immune system.

So if you are one of the many people who do a lot of visual concentration, be sure you check your face muscles every fifteen minutes or so to see if they're tense. And be sure to let your eyes move frequently. Also, use your peripheral vision as often as you can.

BREATH-RELATED SHOULDER ROLLS FOR NECK AND SHOULDER TENSION

One of the main problems that occurs as we sit for long hours at our computers or desks is that our neck and shoulders become very tight and locked into tension patterns that are very difficult to release. This restricts blood and nerve flow to our brain and nervous system and contributes greatly to constricted breathing and an overall sense of stress.

If occasional stretching does not reduce or eliminate this tension, which it sometimes won't, try this very effective exercise to break up the patterns of tension in these areas.[4]

Make sure you're sitting on your chair with your back upright but relaxed. Sense your breathing. Allow your belly to expand on the in-breath and retract on the out-breath. Take several breaths in this way. Now, with your elbows bent and upper arms against your chest, place the fingers of your right hand on the very top of your right shoulder and the fingers of your left hand on the very top of your left shoulder (fig. B.1a).

As you inhale, let your head drop slowly in front of you as you draw your elbows upward in front of you as high as you comfortably can (fig. B.1b). Then, as you exhale, circle your elbows slowly out to

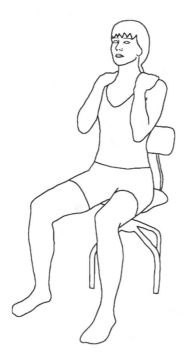

FIGURE B.1a
Breath-related shoulder rolls:
starting position

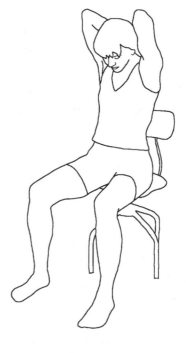

FIGURE B.1b
Breath-related shoulder rolls:
draw elbows up

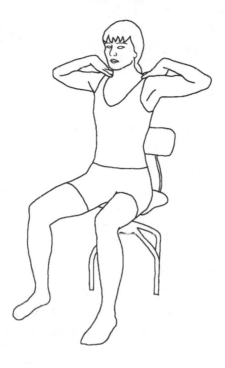

FIGURE B.IC
Breath-related shoulder rolls: circle elbows to sides

the sides (right elbow to the right side and left elbow to the left as in figure B.IC) and back down to the beginning position as you gradually lift your head back to the upright position.

As you do these movements, stay in touch with the movements also taking place in your belly, but do not force your inhalation or exhalation. Let them happen naturally, and be sure they are timed with the simultaneous movement of the head and elbows. Do the exercise as slowly and as evenly as you can. You can do this exercise up to six times, three times a day.

ISOMETRIC EXERCISE WITH BELLY BREATHING FOR NECK TENSION

A tense or stiff neck will cause restrictions in your breathing. If your neck is particularly tense or stiff, try this exercise.[5] Lock your hands (interwoven fingers) behind your head. Keep your head perfectly straight in space as you simultaneously apply equal pressure (don't strain) in opposite directions from your hands and your head. In other words, your locked hands and head push against each other while your head remains motionless. At the same time, have the sense that you are breathing into and out of your belly in a very relaxed and comfortable way. This will help keep your breathing from centering itself in your upper chest. You can do this exercise for up to three minutes at a time. When you finish, pay particular attention to the warmth in your belly and the surge of energy in your head and brain.

EMERGENCY STRESS AND BLOOD PRESSURE REDUCTION EXERCISE

This exercise, which originates from the vast panoply of pranayama exercises and has been discussed by Dr. Andrew Weil in his newsletter,[6] is said by him to be useful for the temporary reduction of blood pressure and stress. I have verified its ability to temporarily reduce blood pressure and stress in many instances and am including my version of it here with a special warning.

Warning

If you have high blood pressure, you must discuss this exercise with your doctor before undertaking it. You should not cease taking any blood pressure medication without the express approval of your doctor.

In general, I do not recommend breath-holding exercises (especially after the in-breath), which this is. Because of the high levels of stress, anxiety, and fear in today's world, many of us hold our breath a lot. Over time, this can have an adverse influence on the diaphragm, which functions best when it is able to move evenly and freely in a coordinated way through its entire range of motion.

Practicing this Exercise

My version of this exercise is easy to practice. Simply inhale through your nose for four counts, hold your breath for seven counts, and exhale through your mouth for eight counts. When you exhale, put the tip of your tongue at the point of the intersection between your upper front teeth and the roof of your mouth, and exhale as though you are blowing out a candle. Let the inhalation come by itself. Don't force it. Start with a set of four complete breaths (each breath is one inhalation and one exhalation) for the first couple of weeks. If you wish you can then gradually work your way up to a set of eight complete breaths over the next couple of weeks. You can do two sets daily on a regular basis.

In doing this exercise, be sure to count evenly through the inhalation, breath holding, and exhalation. You can use your heartbeat (if you can sense it), or a watch, or simply count. Don't use force. Keep your mouth, tongue, chest, back, and belly as relaxed as possible. Remember, this is an extremely powerful breath-control exercise. Except when you need to use it on an emergency basis for your blood pressure, don't do it more than a couple of times a day.

APPENDIX C

Suggested Practice Routines

Daily Breathing Practices: Twenty to Thirty Minutes
Opening Up Your Breathing Spaces: Forty-five to Sixty Minutes
  Twice a Week
Stress-Buster Exercises: Two to Five Minutes
Daily Healing Practices: Ten to Sixty Minutes
Learning to Let Go and Live in the Present Moment: Thirty Minutes
  Daily

ONE SIZE DOES NOT FIT ALL

As I said in the Introduction, "When it comes to breathing, one size does not fit all . . . there is no one set of breathing exercises or practices that is appropriate for everyone." Once you have worked through all the material in this book with full awareness, therefore, it will be up to you to decide which practices, exercises, and meditations are most useful for you at any particular time. In this way, the work you do will be more intimate and relevant, based on your own inner sincerity and awareness and not on some fixed, rigid program. That being said, here are a few suggestions for how you might tailor the exercises and practices in this book in relation to specific situations or time constraints. These are just suggestions. Feel free to add other exercises or practices from the book that you find enjoyable and useful.

DAILY BREATHING PRACTICES: TWENTY TO THIRTY MINUTES

Several of the practices in this book are extremely helpful for your breathing when done on a daily basis. These include:

- Stretching to Open Up Your Breathing Spaces
- Pelvic Circles
- The Bouncing Breath
- Belly Breathing
- The Humming Breath
- Lengthening Your Exhalation and Revitalizing Your Lungs
- The Relaxation Pose
- Conscious Breathing (it is helpful to end your daily session with this practice)

OPENING UP YOUR BREATHING SPACES: FORTY-FIVE TO SIXTY MINUTES TWICE A WEEK

At the heart of free, healthy breathing is the ability of your breath to fully engage all of your breathing spaces. Depending on your posture and breathing habits, as well as on your physical, emotional, and spiritual health, fully opening up your breathing spaces can take many months or even years. It may also require the help of a body worker, osteopath, breathing therapist, and other specialists.

When you have forty-five to sixty minutes available at a time, work with all the practices in Chapter Two: Opening Up the Breathing Spaces of the Body (starting with Following Your Breath) at least twice a week, but more days if possible. You can also add qigong, taiji, or other practices from other disciplines that you find useful for helping to release your breathing restrictions. The key, as always, is to work slowly and gently with full awareness.

STRESS-BUSTER EXERCISES: TWO TO FIVE MINUTES

When you find yourself stressed out and unable to take a full, easy breath, any of the following exercises can help in a safe, comfortable way to disrupt your restricted breathing patterns, temporarily open up your breathing spaces, and thus both relax and energize you.

- Stretching to Open Up Your Breathing Spaces
- Belly Breathing
- The Bouncing Breath
- The Laughing Breath
- The Humming Breath
- Lengthening Your Exhalation and Revitalizing Your Lungs
- A Safe, Simple Exercise for Stress Relief (Appendix B)
- Breathing to Reduce Pain (Appendix B)
- The LA LA LA Practice (Appendix B)

DAILY HEALING PRACTICES: TEN TO SIXTY MINUTES

Because full, natural breathing supports our health and well-being at every level of ourselves, all the practices in the book are helpful both for health maintenance and for healing. The following practices, however, may be especially relevant, depending on your health situation.

- Breathing into a Tight Area in Your Body
- The Laughing Breath
- Conscious Breathing
- The Six Healing Exhalations
- The Smiling Breath

LEARNING TO LET GO AND LIVE IN THE PRESENT MOMENT: THIRTY MINUTES DAILY

Though it may seem paradoxical to specify an amount of time required for learning to let go and live in the present moment, it is not really so. Working with our attention and awareness in the present moment takes practice, and this practice takes time—time in which we can actually experience a more intimate quality of presence. Though all of the practices in the book will support this work if they are done with care and attention, the following practices are especially relevant. Some of these practices require that you set aside thirty minutes of quiet time in your daily life, while others can be done in the midst of your daily activities. For the practices that require special quiet time, you can do a separate one each day. Do not try to do them all in one sitting.

- The Shoulders and Feet Exercise
- Lengthening Your Exhalation and Revitalizing Your Lungs
- Taking Off Your Self-Identity
- Conscious Breathing
- The Breath of the Heart
- Expanding Time
- The Boundless Breath
- A Conscious Standing Practice (Appendix A)
- A Conscious Walking Practice (Appendix A)

Notes

INTRODUCTION

1. See, for example, H. J. Schunemann, et al. "Long-term Predictor of Mortality in the General Population," *Chest* 2000; 118(3) 656–664.
2. Robert Fried, *Breathe Well, Be Well* (New York: John Wiley and Sons, 1999), p. 18.
3. In a visit to my osteopath on a day when my chest felt particularly tight, my breathing suddenly became so free and easy from his hands-on work that I almost didn't recognize myself. Lying on the table, I could sense my chest, as well as my abdomen, expanding and retracting on the in-breath and out-breath spontaneously, effortlessly, and well beyond what was normal for me in a resting posture. In our discussion of this experience, the osteopath told me that my ribs had been locked up and relatively motionless and that this had been impeding my breathing.
4. An earlier version of the meditative practices in Chapter Four was originally offered as an online Internet product called *Boundless Breathing*. Three of these six practices have also appeared in different versions in either my book *The Tao of Natural Breathing* or my audio program, *Breathing as a Metaphor for Living*. Some exercises in the book have been taken from some of the other Internet products that I used to offer, including *Breathing Perspectives* and *Breath Gym*. I have included a variety of new exercises as well as three new meditative practices, and revised and/or expanded those three meditative practices previously published, because I believe that together they are highly appropriate not only for helping to reduce unnecessary tension and stress in today's fast-paced world, but also for putting us in touch with more of the whole of ourselves.
5. I remember once being in a class with Moshe Feldenkrais. We were doing

some floor exercises based on his verbal descriptions. One of the people, who apparently felt he didn't quite understand the exercise, looked up and began to imitate someone else who was doing it. Feldenkrais stopped the whole class and gave us a lecture on why we shouldn't imitate others when doing this work of awareness. He pointed out that it is through our willingness to experiment and to make mistakes that we make new discoveries and that the brain and nervous system learn the most.

CHAPTER ONE:
WAYS OF WORKING WITH YOUR BREATH

1. I have not gone into the principles underlying the powerful methods of holotropic breath work, rebirthing, and so on mainly because they require the ongoing help of experienced guides and even therapists. These are simply not practices that you can undertake on your own.
2. This quotation is from some literature that was handed out during a party I attended to celebrate with Ilse Middendorf her ninetieth birthday, which was held in San Francisco, CA.
3. Candace B. Pert, *Molecules of Emotion* (New York: Scribner, 1997), p. 293.
4. You will find this account in his newsletter *Self Healing* (September 1999), p. 3.
5. I have included my own version of this practice in Appendix B.
6. You can learn more about some of Dr. Konstantin Pavlovich Buteyko's methods, as well as how they are being applied for conditions such as asthma, in *Breathing Free* by Teresa Hale (New York: Harmony Books, 1999). There is also a lot of information about him on the Internet.
7. Buteyko, as represented by his various proponents, even apparently goes so far as to claim that deep breathing is bad for us. Though I believe that the "overbreathing" he associates with deep breathing has nothing actually to do with the real meaning of deep breathing, it is nevertheless an unfortunate claim. In any case, there is a wealth of research from around the world that shows the many benefits of deep breathing for our physical, emotional, and spiritual health.
8. Leonard Laskow, M.D., *Healing with Love: A Breakthrough Mind/Body Medical Program for Healing Yourself and Others* (Mill Valley, CA: Wholeness Press, 1992), p. 61.
9. Ibid, p. 99.
10. Ilse Middendorf, Carl Stough, Mike White, and others have all written or spoken about some of the problems associated with breath holding and excessive tension.

11. From a phone conversation with Mike White in late 2001 regarding this book.

12. Of course, while this outer process of breathing is taking place in our lungs, there is also an inner process taking place in the cells of the brain and body. The cells themselves "inhale" oxygen from the hemoglobin flowing through the body and "exhale" carbon dioxide back into the hemoglobin.

13. See *The Tao of Natural Breathing* for an in-depth discussion of the influence of negative emotions on our breathing.

14. Some people who do aerobics, for example, do so when they are angry or anxious. Though they will certainly get aerobic benefits from this, the anxiety or anger will animate their movements and will actually serve to restrict their breathing muscles and make them work in a less-efficient way.

15. When you move from an emotion of happiness, for example, your breath will generally be fuller than when you move from an emotion of impatience. Impatient movement generally directs your breathing to the top, front part of your chest.

16. Written for this book in April 2002 by Ken Lossing, D.O., San Rafael, CA.

17. Many people with asthma are fast, shallow breathers. Fast shallow breathing does indeed promote the excessive loss of carbon dioxide. What is needed, I believe, is not to breathe less, but to breathe in a slower, more harmonious way, utilizing all the breathing spaces, including one's belly and back. This will reduce "overbreathing," thus ensuring that carbon dioxide levels are maintained at a healthy level, and it will do so in a way that promotes healthy, dynamic breathing.

18. Sleep apnea is a condition in which a person's breathing stops many times an hour, without the person knowing it. In a study reported in the *New England Journal of Medicine* (2000, 342(19), 1378–1384), University of Wisconsin researchers, who followed more than seven hundred people for some four to eight years, found that those people who had the worst sleep apnea at the beginning of the study were the ones most likely to later develop high blood pressure. Though doctors are not sure of the causal mechanism, Paul E. Peppard, of the university's preventative-medicine department, stated that reduced oxygen in the blood might well put the sympathetic nervous system, the part of the nervous system that reacts to stress and prepares the body for action, into "high alert." According to the study, severe sleep apnea can triple a person's chances of developing high blood pressure, while moderate apnea, defined as less than fifteen interruptions an hour, can double a person's chances, and mild sleep apnea, defined as fewer that five interruptions an hour, can increase a person's chances by 40 percent. People with sleep apnea are likely to snore loudly and wake up feeling tired.

19. Andre van Lysebeth, *Pranayama: The Yoga of Breathing* (London: Unwin Paperbacks, 1988), p. 64.
20. This is related to "ultradian rhythms," long observed by medical science, in which the nostrils alternately become more open and more congested every ninety to one hundred twenty minutes. When the left nostril is more open, the right hemisphere of the brain is generally more dominant; when the right nostril is more open, the left hemisphere is generally more dominant. One can intentionally open a nostril that is more congested and thus make the other hemisphere more active by lying down on one's side with the congested nostril above and continuing to breathe through the nose. As I pointed out in *The Tao of Natural Breathing*, if one is feeling out of sorts or has a headache, lying on one's side with the congested nostril above for fifteen or twenty minutes can often bring relief. Curiously, the advice recounted by Lysebeth to sleep in such a way that we breathe mainly through the right nostril seems to fly in the face of the idea that it would be more beneficial to promote the action of the parasympathetic nervous system during sleep, which would seemingly necessitate lying on one's right side.
21. For further insights on the breath-related effects of such common bodywork techniques as skin pulling, tapping, and pressure, see *Ways to Better Breathing*, by Carola Speads.
22. Michael White, for instance, has developed a highly effective hands-on approach that he uses to help people with breathing problems of many kinds, including asthma and emphysema.
23. From an article by Magda Proskauer, "The Therapeutic Value of Certain Breathing Techniques," in Charles Garfield, ed., *Rediscovery of the Body: A Psychosomatic View of Life and Death* (New York: Dell Publishing Company, 1977), p. 27.
24. In his book *Dr. Breath: The Story of Breathing Coordination*, Carl Stough recounts his discovery of how counting quickly out loud from one to ten during exhalation over and over again (as long as one can do so comfortably) can transform the tone, strength, and functioning of the diaphragm and help coordinate all of the breathing muscles. He used this approach, along with various hands-on techniques, to help many people, including emphysema patients, singers, and Olympic athletes.
25. For instance, take a look at some of the essays in *Music: Physician for Times to Come*, an anthology edited by Don Campbell.
26. Your blood pressure goes up when you talk and down when you listen, says James L. Lynch in his book *A Cry Unheard: New Insights into the Medical Consequences of Loneliness* (Baltimore: Bancroft Press, 2000). According to Lynch, a Baltimore psychologist, for those people with hypertension or who lead quiet, lonely lives, too much talking can be lethal, and the risk goes up, he says, as people get older.
    It is my view that however gregarious we may be, too much talking

(especially if we are also talking too fast) can have a negative influence on our breathing, especially if we don't breathe well to begin with. Too much talking can disharmonize the movement of our breathing muscles, alter the oxygen/carbon dioxide balance in the body, and promote hyperventilation, which can make us feel anxious, worried, uptight, and so on. Over time, too much talking can condition the diaphragm to move in even more constricted, staccato ways, as we breathe through our mouth while struggling for breath in the middle of our sentences. This means that the diaphragm will not be able to function rhythmically and efficiently in helping to empty the lungs, massage our internal organs, and promote lymph flow. If you are in a profession that requires a lot of talking, one thing you can try is slowing down your speech, make it more rhythmical and steady, and, when you're not talking, breathe when possible through your nose. You can and should also practice breathing more from your belly as you speak, and make sure that you keep breathing when you talk. Whenever possible, don't continue talking when you are almost out of breath; simply pause and inhale before continuing.

27. Researchers at the Karolinska Hospital in Sweden found that nitric oxide levels in the sinuses were fifteen times higher when people were humming than when they were breathing normally. Nitric oxide is instrumental in dilating capillary beds and increasing blood flow. The researchers also found that when people hummed there was a 98 percent gas exchange between the nasal passages and the sinuses. During normal exhalation the gas exchange dropped to 4 percent. To understand the significance of this, it is important to realize that bacteria grow most effectively in an environment in which there is poor circulation and a poor exchange of gases. This research was reported in the *American Journal of Respiratory Critical Care Medicine* (2002: 166: 144–45).

28. See, for example, *On a Single Breath: A Lost Interpretation of the Lord's Prayer*, by Sir Paul Dukes. In this account of some meetings with G. I. Gurdjieff (known then to him as Prince Ozay), Dukes discusses Gurdjieff's statement to him that the Lord's Prayer was meant to be chanted on a single note during a single breath, as well as some of the important reasons for this.

29. One finds a wonderful example of this simultaneous work of chanting and listening in the *Harmonic Awareness* workshops given by David Hykes, founder of the Harmonic Choir.

30. I developed this simple practice as a result of my work with David Hykes, harmonic sound pioneer.

31. It is extremely important not to continue trying to hum or make other sounds when you've run out of air. Doing so on a consistent basis will weaken your diaphragm and undermine the coordination of your breathing muscles.

CHAPTER TWO:
OPENING UP THE BREATHING
SPACES OF THE BODY

1. It is important to realize that every unnecessary tension uses energy in an unproductive way. Breathing that is labored because of unnecessary tensions and constrictions in the diaphragm, ribs, back, stomach, and so on wastes our very life force. The release of these tensions and constrictions will bring us more energy, energy that would otherwise be consumed by the very process of breathing itself.
2. For dealing with neck and shoulder tension, try Breath Related Shoulder Rolls for Neck and Shoulder Tension and Isometric Exercise with Belly Breathing for Neck Tension in Appendix B.
3. From "Breathing Therapy," by Magda Proskauer, in Herbert A. Otto and John Mann, eds., *Ways of Growth: Approaches to Expanding Awareness* (New York: Viking Press, 1971) p. 27.
4. This quotation appeared in the February 2002 edition (Volume 9, No. 8) of *Alternatives for the Health-Conscious Individual*, a monthly newsletter written by Dr. David C. Williams and published by Mountain Home Publishing in Potomac, MD.
5. This exercise, as well as Raise Palm and Lift Knee, comes from a set of practices that I teach called *Liangong in 18 Exercises*. I was given permission to teach this set of practices by Dr. Wang Shan Long, a qigong master from China.

CHAPTER THREE:
THE METAPHYSICAL BREATH

1. Len Saputo, M.D., and Nancy Faass, M.S.W., eds., *Boosting Immunity: Creating Wellness Naturally* (Novato, CA: New World Library, 2002), p. 230.
2. Karlfried Graf von Durckheim, *The Way of Transformation: Daily Life as Spiritual Practice* (London: George Allen and Unwin, 1971), p. 38.
3. In working with others using Chi Nei Tsang (internal organ chi massage) and various breath therapy techniques, I have put my hands on hundreds of bellies. In many cases, people's bellies were so tight and immobile that they were not able to expand and contract with each breath. As I explain in *The Tao of Natural Breathing*, tight bellies are caused by many things, including negative emotions and trauma.
4. Our day-to-day lung volume depends on several factors, including genet-

ics, environmental factors, disease, the coordination of our breathing muscles, the degree to which the diaphragm can move through its full range of potential motion, and the difference in chest circumference between exhalation and inhalation. On his Web site, Michael Grant White discusses research that shows that a larger differential in chest circumference between exhalation and inhalation is statistically associated with greater longevity.

5. *The Tao of Natural Breathing*, p. 119.

6. According to Gurdjieff, "identification" with our thoughts and feelings is one of the main obstacles for anyone who is searching for wholeness. You can learn more about this fascinating subject in the book *In Search of the Miraculous* by P. D. Ouspensky.

7. This practice is an adaptation of a practice I learned from Advaita Vedanta master Jean Klein in various workshops and retreats.

CHAPTER FOUR: GOING DEEPER—PRACTICES AND MEDITATIONS FOR SELF-EXPLORATION

1. Mantak Chia teaches the six healing sounds in conjunction with specific postures and movements. For the purposes of this book, I have included postures and movements for only one of the sounds. If you would like to learn the postures and movements that Mantak Chia teaches in relation to these sounds, you can read his book *Transform Stress into Vitality*.

2. See *The Tao of Natural Breathing* for some of the research related to how intentional smiling influences "regional brain activity," as well as for some ideas about how it alters our emotions.

3. This practice is a shortened and modified version of the "Inner Smile" meditation first brought to the West by Taoist master Mantak Chia. This version puts more emphasis on the breath. A slightly different version of this practice appears in my book *The Tao of Natural Breathing*.

4. P. D. Ouspensky, *In Search of the Miraculous*.

5. You can find a wonderful exposition of the work of "inner dissolving" in the two-volume set of books by Taoist master Bruce Kumar Frantzis, entitled *Relaxing into Your Being* and *The Great Stillness*.

APPENDIX A:
OTHER CORE TEACHINGS AND PRACTICES

1. Barry Sears, *The Age Free Zone* (New York: Regan Books/Harper Collins, 1999), p. 21.
2. Peg Jordan, *The Fitness Instinct* (Emmaus, PA: Rodale Press, 1999), pp. 38–40.
3. From J. A. O'Krey, "Oxygen Uptake and Ventilatory Effects of an External Nasal Dilator During Ergonomatry" in *Medicine and Science in Sports and Medicine* 32 (2000): 1491–1495.
4. Here, again, what and how much we eat can also have a powerful influence on our aerobic capacity, which depends in large part on the diameter of the capillaries around our lung tissue. The larger the diameter of the capillaries, the more oxygen will be transferred to the red blood cells. According to Barry Sears in *The Age Free Zone* (New York: Regan Books/Harper Collins: 1999, p. 21), elevated insulin produces excessive amounts of hormones called vasoconstrictors that decrease the diameter of the capillaries and thus impede oxygen flow to the cells. When our insulin is in the normal range, we produce more vasodilators, which actually increase the diameter of the capillaries, thus facilitating oxygen transfer. What's more, says Sears, oxygen transfer depends on "the flexibility of your red blood cells." Certain hormones in the body either make it easier or harder for the red blood cells "to contort or deform themselves as they squeeze through the capillaries. . . ." Elevated insulin produces hormones that make our red blood cells less flexible and thus less able to bring oxygen to the cells.
5. Candace B. Pert, *Molecules of Emotion*, (New York: Scribner, 1997) p. 296.

APPENDIX B:
HELPFUL BREATH-RELATED EXERCISES
FOR DAILY LIVING

1. In the all-too-common caricature of someone trying to take a deep breath, we see a person with lifted shoulders, an overly expanded chest, an arched back, and a belly that is pulled tightly inward. This is actually a picture of someone taking an extremely shallow breath.
2. One study, for example, appeared on bmj.com, the general medical journal Web site *British Medical Journal* 323 (December 22, 2001) (7327): 1446–1449. Entitled "Effect of Rosary Prayer and Yoga Mantras on Autonomic Cardiovascular Rhythms: Comparative Study," this study also

found that a breathing rate of six breaths a minute is optimal. The contributors to this research included the following internal medicine and cardiovascular professors and physicians: Luciano Bernardi, associate professor of internal medicine, Dipartimento di Medicina Interna, University of Pavia, 27100 Pavia, Italy; Peter Sleight, professor, Department of Cardiovascular Medicine, John Radcliffe Hospital, Oxford OX3 9DU; Gabriele Bandinelli, physician, Simone Cencetti, physician, Lamberto Fattorini, physician, and Alfonso Lagi, physician, all at Dipartimento di Medicina Interna, Unitá Ospedaliera S. Maria Nuova, 50100 Florence, Italy; and Johanna Wdowczyc-Szulc, assistant professor of cardiology, Department of Cardiology, University of Gdansk, 80–211 Gdansk, Poland.

3. This discussion of the influence of breathing on the PAG, including the two brief quotations, is from Dharma Singh Khalsa, M.D., and Cameron Stauth, *Meditation as Medicine* (New York: Pocket Books, 2001), pp. 61–62.

4. This practice is adapted and expanded from an osteopathic exercise found in *Dr. Fulford's Touch of Life*, p. 180, Exercise 6.

5. Isometric exercises such as this one are used by many health care practitioners, including osteopaths. When I was a child, my father showed me this exercise (without the belly breathing) to strengthen my neck. You can find a similar version of this exercise, without the belly breathing, in *Dr. Fulford's Touch of Life*, p. 184, Exercise 8.

6. *Self Healing*, (Watertown, MA: Thorne Communications, Sept. 1999, p. 3).

For Further Exploration

Campbell, Don, ed. *Music: Physician for Times to Come.* Wheaton, IL: Quest Books, 2000. Informative essays by scientists, musicians, music therapists, and spiritual explorers on the healing power of sound.

——. *The Roar of Silence: Healing Powers of Breath, Tone and Music.* Wheaton, IL: The Theosophical Publishing House, 1994. An inspiring exploration of sound and vibration, with excellent toning and chanting exercises.

Chia, Mantak. *Transform Stress into Vitality.* Huntington, NJ: Healing Tao Books, 1985. An excellent introduction to the Taoist practices of the Inner Smile, Six Healing Sounds, and Microcosmic Orbit.

Dukes, Sir Paul. *On a Single Breath: A Lost Interpretation of the Lord's Prayer, an account of some meetings with George Ivanovich Gurdjieff.* Denville, NJ: Indications Press, 1996. This extraordinary little book touches on the esoteric relationship of breath and prayer.

Durckheim, Karlfried Graf von. *The Way of Transformation: Daily Life as Spiritual Practice.* London: George Allen and Unwin, 1971. Written by the author of the classic *Hara: The Vital Center of Man*, this book explores the intimate relationship of body and soul in the search for transcendental freedom and essential being.

Dychtwald, Ken. *BodyMind.* Los Angeles: Jeremy P. Tarcher, 1977. A practical and illuminating investigation of the ways in which our bodies (and breath) reflect our emotions, traumas, and other life experiences.

Farhi, Donna. *The Breathing Book: Good Health and Vitality through Essential Breath Work.* New York: Henry Holt and Company, 1996. This comprehensive book, written by an internationally known yoga teacher, provides knowledge, insights, and exercises that can help you breathe in a healthier way.

Feldenkrais, Moshe. *Awareness through Movement: Easy-to-Do Health Exercises to Improve Posture, Vision, Imagination, and Personal Awareness.* San Francisco: Harper San Francisco, 1991. This is a must-read book for anyone interested in movement, posture, and somatic awareness.

Frantzis, Bruce. *Relaxing into Your Being*. Fairfax, CA: Clarity Press, 1998, and *The Great Stillness*. Fairfax, CA: Clarity Press, 1999. These important books by a worldwide teacher of qigong, internal martial arts, and meditation explain the essence and practical techniques of the water method of Taoist meditation, including the process of inner dissolving.

Fried, Robert. *Breathe Well, Be Well*. New York: John Wiley and Sons, 1999. This highly respected book, written by the head of the respiratory psychophysiology laboratory at Hunter College, offers helpful information on many aspects of breathing, including "the hyperventilation syndrome" and the relationship of nutrition to breathing.

Fulford, Robert C., D.O., with Gene Stone. *Dr. Fulford's Touch of Life: The Healing Power of the Life Force*. New York: Pocket Books, 1996. One of the great osteopaths, Fulford spent some sixty years treating patients whom conventional medicine could not help. This book is filled with helpful insights about healing.

Hendricks, Gay. *Conscious Breathing: Breathwork for Health, Stress Release, and Personal Mastery*. New York: Bantam Books, 1995. A highly respected, informative book on the relationship of breathing to many aspects of our lives. Includes many great exercises to help us breathe more fully and naturally.

Huang, Jane., trans., in collaboration with Michael Wurmbrand. *The Primordial Breath: An Ancient Chinese Way of Prolonging Life through Breath Control*, Volumes 1 and 2. Torrance, CA: Original Books, 1987. Treatises on breathing (in English) from the Taoist Canon, the Tao Tsang.

Hykes, David. *Harmonic Awareness/Harmonic Chant, Volume 1: Music, Meditation, Harmonization* (teaching CD). Hykes, founder of the Harmonic Choir, also offers many Harmonic Chant CDs, including *Hearing Solar Winds*, *Rainbow Dances*, and *Breath of the Heart*. Hear samples of his extraordinary CDs or purchase them through the Harmonic World Web site at http://www.harmonicworld.com.

Jordan, Peg. *The Fitness Instinct*. Emmaus, PA: Rodale Press, Inc., 1999. A wonderful guide to discovering your own individual approach to fitness, written by the founder and editor-in chief of *American Fitness Magazine*.

Kahn, Hazrat Inayat. *The Mysticism of Sound and Music*. Boston and London: Shambhala, 1996. The great classic on the mystery and divine nature of sound and music.

Klein, Jean. *Who Am I: The Sacred Quest*. Longmead, England: Element Books, 1988. A powerful exploration into our true nature by a modern Advaita Vedanta master.

Lewis, Dennis. *The Tao of Natural Breathing: For Health, Well-Being and Inner Growth*. San Francisco: Mountain Wind Publishing, 1996. A fascinating journey into the physiology, psychology, and spirituality of authentic breathing, with numerous exercises.

———. *Breathing as a Metaphor for Living: Teachings and Exercises on Complete and Natural Breathing*. Boulder, CO: Sounds True, 1998. Two-cassette audio program. Includes ideas, insights, and meditative practices that can help you discover your own authentic breath.

Middendorf, Ilse. *The Perceptible Breath: A Breathing Science*. Paderborn, Germany: Junfermann-Verlag, 1990.Written by one of the world's foremost explorers of the breath, this is a primary resource for anyone interested in learning more about breathing.

Ouspensky, P. D. *In Search of the Miraculous*. New York: Harcourt, Brace, and World, 1949. The classic on the ideas and methods of G. I. Gurdjieff, the extraordinary spiritual master and teacher who bridged East and West and showed that awakening from our sleep must be the number one priority for those of us interested in real being.

Rama, Swami, Rudolph Ballentine, M.D., and Alan Hymes, M.D., *Science of Breath*. Honesdale, PA: Himalayan Institute, 1981. Brings together some of the important scientific discoveries of the West and experiential discoveries of the East with regard to breath.

Speads, Carola. *Ways to Better Breathing*. Rochester, VT: Healing Arts Press, 1992. One of the best books on breathing currently available.

Stough, Carl and Reece Stough. *Dr. Breath: The Story of Breathing Coordination*. New York: The Stough Institute, 1981. A fascinating account of Stough's discovery of the importance of "breathing coordination" for everyone from athletes and singers to those suffering from emphysema.

Hanh, Thich Nhat. *Breathe! You Are Alive: Sutra on the Full Awareness of Breathing*. Berkeley: Parallax Press, 1960. Shows how the conscious breathing methods taught by the Buddha can be practiced today.

Todd, Mabel Elsworth. *The Thinking Body*. New York: Dance Horizons, 1973. A profound study of the complex mechanisms of breathing, locomotion, and mechanical balance in the human organism, with the aim of understanding the real meaning of relaxation.

Tolle, Eckhart. *The Power of Now: A Guide to Spiritual Enlightenment*. Novato, CA: New World Library, 1999. Tolle helps us return with full presence to the only place and time where awakening is possible: right here, right now.

White, Michael Grant. *Secrets of Optimal Natural Breathing*. Waynesville, NC: Optimal Breathing Press, 2003. Mike White is well known as a hands-on breathing work practitioner who has helped numerous people, including singers, athletes, and those with breath-related medical problems. You can learn more at http://www.breathing.com.

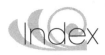

Index